CHRONIC COUGH

CHRONIC COUGH

Thomas L. Carroll, MD

PLURAL PUBLISHING
INC.

PLURAL PUBLISHING
INC.

5521 Ruffin Road
San Diego, CA 92123

Email: information@pluralpublishing.com
Website: http://www.pluralpublishing.com

Typeset in 11/13 Palatino by Flanagan's Publishing Services, Inc.
Printed in the United States of America by Integrated Books International

Library of Congress Cataloging-in-Publication Data

Names: Carroll, Thomas L. (Thomas Leigh), editor.
Title: Chronic cough / [edited by] Thomas L. Carroll.
Other titles: Chronic cough (Carroll)
Description: San Diego, CA : LOGO Plural Publishing, [2019] | Includes bibliographical references and index.
Identifiers: LCCN 2018055141 | ISBN 9781635500707 (alk. paper) | ISBN 1635500702 (alk. paper)
Subjects: | MESH: Cough | Chronic Disease
Classification: LCC RC741.5 | NLM WF 143 | DDC 616.2—dc23
LC record available at https://lccn.loc.gov/2018055141

CONTENTS

Preface *vii*
Contributors *ix*

1 Overview of Chronic Cough and Its Impact on Health Care **1**
Seth H. Dailey and Johnny P. Mai

2 Cough-Variant Asthma and Related Diseases **21**
Nicole L. Grossman and Christopher H. Fanta

3 Sinonasal Disease and Allergy as an Etiology of Chronic Cough **39**
Alice Z. Maxfield and Benjamin S. Bleier

4 Reflux Disease **65**
Matthew P. Partain and Jonathan M. Bock

5 Basic Science Considerations for Laryngopharyngeal Reflux (LPR) **81**
Miles Klimara and Nikki Johnston

6 Neurogenic Cough **97**
John Paul Giliberto and Albert Merati

7 Dysphagia in Chronic Cough **117**
Mark A. Fritz, Debra M. Suiter, and Gregory N. Postma

8 Cough Management: The Speech-Language Pathologist's Role in the Treatment of Chronic Cough **143**
Hadas Golan and Chandler C. Thompson

9 A Treatment Paradigm for Refractory Chronic Cough: Putting It All Together in a Quaternary Cough Referral Practice **173**
Thomas L. Carroll

10 Chronic Cough: Future Directions **187**
Adrianna C. Shembel, Paul E. Kwak, and Milan R. Amin

Index *201*

PREFACE

The diagnosis and treatment of chronic cough is a moving target but one, thankfully, that is moving in the right direction. Empiric treatments are giving way to objective testing. Research drives new therapeutics and testing modalities. Patients are more frequently being treated successfully after decades of coughing through diagnostic advances and multidisciplinary collaboration. Chronic cough is being recognized more as a symptom of an underlying issue rather than as a primary diagnosis with an unclear etiology.

This book was proposed and is now realized as a clinical resource for practitioners who see and treat patients with chronic cough. It is intended as a reference for any clinician in practice or training who wants to feel more confident in their understanding, workup, and treatment of this symptom. It will especially appeal to those residents, advanced practice providers, and physicians in the fields of family practice, internal medicine, otolaryngology, pulmonology, gastroenterology, and speech-language pathology. Multiple experts from backgrounds in otolaryngology, including laryngology and rhinology, pulmonology, molecular and cellular pathology, and speech-language pathology contributed to this book.

This book's 10 chapters are designed to cover the basics of what we know, what we don't know, and what we are discovering about chronic cough. In addition, the chapters offer a platform for each chapter's authors to "think outside the box" and speak directly to the reader on their given subject matter and cover controversial or less-conventional ideas surrounding chronic cough. The book begins with an overview of chronic cough that sets the stage for the remaining chapters. After covering the highest-yield topics on the subject, the penultimate chapter puts together the previous topics as a treatment paradigm that intends to help approach a patient with refractory chronic cough in a quaternary referral setting and make headway to symptom relief.

There is no one algorithm to treating chronic cough, but there are ways to organize one's approach and this should be the goal. The final chapter of this book is an expanded version of "thinking outside of the box." It will introduce the reader to causes of chronic cough that are not commonly considered by clinicians outside of laryngology and speech-language pathology but are emerging as real possibilities for therapy.

The pendulum is swinging away from 30 years of empiric acid suppression medical therapy to more objective reflux and motility testing for pepsin-mediated laryngopharyngeal reflux disease. Considerations of novel therapeutics and diagnostic modalities for asthma are evolving and prompting consideration of other pulmonary diagnoses for chronic cough patients. Revelations in the etiology and effects of sinonasal disease and allergy as a contributor to chronic cough are continuing to impress upon us a need for more information. The role of speech-language pathologists in the behavioral management of chronic cough is growing and proving critical. Dysphagia and dysmotility are often underappreciated causes of chronic cough and are more recently being brought into focus. Primary vocal fold pathologies and neurolaryngeal disorders are waiting to be understood in more complexity to help chronic cough patients that have an indeterminate etiology for their cough.

—Thomas L. Carroll, MD

CONTRIBUTORS

Milan R. Amin, MD
Associate Professor
Director, NYU Voice Center
Clinical Vice Chair
Department of Otolaryngology—Head and Neck Surgery
New York University School of Medicine
New York, New York
Chapter 10

Benjamin S. Bleier, MD, FARS, FACS
Associate Professor
Harvard Medical School
Massachusetts Eye and Ear Infirmary
Boston, Massachusetts
Chapter 3

Jonathan M. Bock, MD, FACS
Associate Professor
Division of Laryngology and Professional Voice
Department of Otolaryngology and Communication Sciences
Medical College of Wisconsin
Milwaukee, Wisconsin
Chapter 4

Thomas L. Carroll, MD
Assistant Professor
Department of Otolaryngology
Harvard Medical School
Director, Brigham and Women's Voice Program
Brigham and Women's Hospital
Boston, Massachusetts
Chapter 9

Seth H. Dailey, MD
Professor of Surgery
Chief, Section of Laryngology and Voice Surgery
Program Director, Laryngology Fellowship
Division of Otolaryngology—Head and Neck Surgery
University of Wisconsin-Madison Hospital
Madison, Wisconsin
Chapter 1

Christopher H. Fanta, MD
Member
Pulmonary and Critical Care Medicine Division
Brigham and Women's Hospital
Director
Partners Asthma Center
Professor of Medicine
Harvard Medical Center
Boston, Massachusetts
Chapter 2

Mark A. Fritz, MD
Assistant Professor
Department of Otolaryngology—Head and Neck Surgery
University of Kentucky College of Medicine
Lexington, Kentucky
Chapter 7

John Paul Giliberto, MD
Assistant Professor
University of Washington
Seattle, Washington
Chapter 6

Hadas Golan, MS, CCC-SLP
Speech-Language Pathologist
Department of Otolaryngology
Boston University Medical Center
Boston, Massachusetts
Chapter 8

Nicole L. Grossman, MD
Clinical Assistant Professor
Tufts University School of Medicine
Senior Staff Physician
Pulmonary and Critical Care Medicine
Lahey Hospital and Medical Center
Burlington, Massachusetts
Chapter 2

Nikki Johnston, PhD
Associate Professor
Department of Otolaryngology and Communication Sciences
Department of Microbiology and Immunology
Medical College of Wisconsin

Milwaukee, Wisconsin
Chapter 5

Miles Klimara, BA
MD Student
Medical College of Wisconsin
Milwaukee, Wisconsin
Chapter 5

Paul E. Kwak, MD, MM, MSc
Assistant Professor
Department of Otolaryngology—Head and Neck Surgery
NYU Langone Medical Center
New York, New York
Chapter 10

Johnny P. Mai, MD
Fellow
University of Wisconsin-Madison
Madison, Wisconsin
Chapter 1

Alice Z. Maxfield, MD
Division of Otolaryngology
Brigham and Women's Hospital
Department of Otolaryngology
Harvard Medical School
Boston, Massachusetts
Chapter 3

Albert Merati, MD, FACS
Professor and Chief, Laryngology
Department of Otolaryngology—Head and Neck Surgery
University of Washington School of Medicine
Adjunct Professor, Department of Speech and Hearing Sciences
Adjunct Professor, School of Music
University of Washington
Seattle, Washington
Chapter 6

Matthew P. Partain, MD
Resident Physician
Department of Otolaryngology and Communication Sciences
Medical College of Wisconsin
Milwaukee, Wisconsin
Chapter 4

Gregory N. Postma, MD
Director, Center for Voice, Airway, and Swallowing Disorders
Professor and Vice Chairman, Department of Otolaryngology
Medical College of Georgia
Augusta University
Augusta, Georgia
Chapter 7

Adrianna C. Shembel, PhD, CCC-SLP
Postdoctoral Research Fellow
NYU Voice Center, Department of Otolaryngology—Head and Neck Surgery
NYU Langone Medical Center
NYU School of Medicine
New York, New York
Chapter 10

Debra M. Suiter, PhD, CCC-SLP, BCS-S
Associate Professor
University of Kentucky
Lexington, Kentucky
Chapter 7

Chandler C. Thompson, DMA, MS, CCC-SLP
Speech-Language Pathologist/Professional Voice
Sean Parker Institute for the Voice
Staff Associate, Department of Otolaryngology
Weill Cornell Medical College
New York, New York
Chapter 8

This book is dedicated to my wife, Kyle, and my two sons Grayson and Davis.
I am immensely fortunate to have your love and support in my life.
I would also like to thank all of my teachers and mentors who instilled in
me an interest and ongoing passion for laryngology, especially
Drs. Mona Abaza, Priya Krishna, Libby Smith, and Clark Rosen.

1

OVERVIEW OF CHRONIC COUGH AND ITS IMPACT ON HEALTH CARE

Seth H. Dailey and Johnny P. Mai

INTRODUCTION TO CHRONIC COUGH

Coughing is the act of rapidly expelling air from the lungs accompanied by a sharp audible sound.[1] Cough is an essential protective function, serving to clear the airway of debris and allowing for continued gas exchange in the lungs. In this protective role, cough prevents life-threatening complications. In an extreme example, pneumonia is known to be the leading cause of mortality in patients with spinal cord injuries where motor nerve paralysis leads to absent cough.[2] Cough can be a volitional action, but more often is an involuntary response to a chemical or environmental stimulus. Despite cough's critical role in airway clearance, persistent cough in the absence of an appropriate stimulus can become pathologic.

Cough is classified as acute, subacute, and chronic based on the duration of cough. An acute cough is one lasting less than 4 weeks and is often secondary to a viral etiology. A cough persisting for 8 weeks or more is defined as chronic, with the interval in between deemed subacute. Albeit arbitrary, this duration is agreed upon by both American and European task forces.[3,4]

The goal of this chapter is to introduce the reader to common causes of chronic cough. Treatment of chronic cough will be discussed only as it pertains to diagnosis. In-depth discussion on treatment of cough is discussed in chapters to follow.

In addition to framing the discussion for subsequent chapters on the various causes and diagnosis of cough, this chapter presents the economic impact of chronic cough. Above all else, this chapter intends to relate this organic pathology back to the patients treated for the condition. By emphasizing the human toll of chronic cough, the purpose of this text is to educate the wide array of practitioners who treat chronic cough for the benefit of their patients.

PHYSIOLOGY OF COUGH

Pathophysiology of Cough

A reflex is defined as an involuntary or nearly instantaneous movement in response to a stimulus.[5] As defined, cough is indeed a reflex serving to clear the tracheal bronchial tree for gas exchange. Cough, unlike other human reflexes such as pupillary light or palmar grasp reflex, is critical for the preservation of life.

The physiologic basis of cough is broken into four distinct phases defined by distinct actions within the phase. Inspiration to fill the lungs is the first action of cough. In the second phase, subglottic pressure increases as there is compression of air against a closed glottis. The third action is marked by the explosive opening of the glottis, leading to rapid increase in airflow. During this phase, the rapid airflow moving through the airway causes a distinctive acoustic emission, which is the hallmark "cough." The sound of a cough is universally recognized and is used to differentiate between other similar expiratory respiratory efforts such as sneezing and throat clearing.[6] The final phase is the restorative phase, in which a final resting breath is taken. The act of coughing is an extraordinary physiologic event capable of producing intrathoracic pressured measured up to 300 mm Hg and airspeed up to 500 miles per hour.[7,8] This particularly violent response can result in urinary and fecal incontinence, pneumothorax, syncope, and even broken ribs.

Neurophysiology of Cough

To understand how cough becomes pathologic, it is useful to understand the neurophysiology of cough in its normative state.

In its essence, cough can be broken down into three constituents: input, processing, and output. The cough reflex involves stimulation of the afferent limb of the cough reflex, then transmission of the stimulation to the cortical cough center and, finally, the efferent pathway, which causes the muscles of expiration to contract, producing cough.

As a caveat, much of what is known about the neuropathophysiology of cough has been inferred through studying animal models, primarily the guinea pig, rather than in vivo human studies. Therefore, despite extensive studies, there is still considerable debate concerning the exact neural sensory mechanism of cough.

Airway sensory nerves originate within either the nodose or jugular vagal ganglia,[9,10] as evident by the fact that a vagotomy or local anesthesia applied to the vagus nerve will abolish the cough reflex.[11,12] The nerve terminals can have endings either in the pulmonary airway and parenchyma or in the extrapulmonary airway, including the carina, trachea, and large bronchi. There is currently no classification schema that neatly characterizes airway afferent nerves given the degree of heterogeneity within the group. This being said, there is consensus that within primary afferent cough fibers, there are nociceptors stimulated by chemical irritants and others stimulated through mechanical means, forming a division where afferents are divided by their physiologic responsiveness to stimuli.

Stretch receptors are well-described intrapulmonary afferents stimulated by mechanical means. When activated by changes in lung volume, airway edema, or smooth muscle constriction, stretch receptor afferents within the lower tracheobronchial tree and parenchyma conduct action potentials at 10 to 20 m/s to cell bodies located in the inferior nodose ganglion. Stretch receptors are further divided into rapid adapting receptors and slowly adapting receptors. The former are more active in the dynamic phase of the respiratory cycle and the latter are more active throughout the respiratory cycle. Stretch receptors help regulate the respiratory cycle, but their role in cough remains uncertain.[13]

A third type of receptor sensitive to mechanical stimulation was first described by Widdicombe in 1954.[14] Unlike stretch receptors, these fibers are found exclusively in the extrapulmonary airway and adapt to punctate mechanical stimuli rather than stretch stimuli. These receptors precipitate an action potential in myelinated vagal afferents at a much slower velocity of 5 m/s, arguing to the uniqueness of these receptors from stretch receptors. Since the first description, the receptors have been eponymously referred to as Widdicombe receptors, then irritant receptors, but are now commonly referred to simply as cough receptors.

Chemical receptors, as the name would suggest, are relatively nonresponsive to mechanical stimulation, requiring 100 times the threshold required for mechanoreceptors. Instead, chemical receptors are sensitive to mediators found during inflammation, irritation, and changes in pH. Customarily, chemical nociceptors are defined by the presence of the ion channel transient receptor potential vanilloid 1 (TRPV1). The TRPV1 receptor binds capsaicin, the active component in chili pepper extracts and a known potent tussigenic agent. The binding affinity of TRPV1 is increased with mediators found during inflammation including bradykinins, prostaglandins, adenosine, and serotonin, as well irritants including nicotine and ozone. An overexpression of TRPV1 can be seen in chronic cough patients.[15]

Chemoreceptors are stereotypically associated with C-fiber afferents, which are classified by their action potential conduction velocity, ranging from 1 to 2 m/ sec.[16] Though C-fibers are most common type of afferent associated with chemoreceptors, afferents with a conduction velocity of 6 m/s, known as alpha-delta afferents, have been shown to conduct action potentials from chemoreceptors.[9]

Table 1–1 provides a summary of the thoracic and extrathoracic afferents that have been associated with cough.

From one's personal experience with volitional cough and conscious cough suppression, it should be clear there is a layer of cortical control in the physiology of cough. Located in the caudal brainstem, the central cough generator receives the vagal afferents via the nucleus tractus solitarius. The ability of cough to undergo central processing is also demonstrated in the efficacy of placebo therapy, which often decreases cough.

COMMON CAUSES OF CHRONIC COUGH

The following discussion serves as a precursory introduction to familiarize the reader to common causes of chronic cough. In-depth appraisal of each etiology is included in subsequent chapters. Furthermore, although the following descriptions discuss common etiologies of chronic cough as

Table 1–1. Vagal Afferents of the Thoracic and Extrathoracic Airway

Stretch Receptors	Cough (Widdicombe) Receptors	Chemoreceptors
Location Intrapulmonary	**Location** Extrapulmonary	**Location** Extrapulmonary & Intrapulmonary
Conduction Speed 10–20 m/s	**Conduction Speed** 5 m/s	**Conduction Speed** C-fibers 1–2 m/s Aδ fibers 6 m/s
Stimulus Rapid Adapting Dynamic Respiration Slow Adapting Static Respiration	**Stimulus** Punctate Mechanical	**Stimulus** Bradykinins, prostaglandins, adenosine, serotonin, pH, capsaicin

singular entities, it is paramount for the reader to appreciate the multifactorial nature of chronic cough. As up to 93% of troublesome coughs are multifactorial, recognition of this salient concept mitigates delay in diagnosis as well as both clinician and patient frustration.[17]

Asthma

Asthma as a source of chronic cough should always be in the differential. Asthmatic patients classically present with wheezing, dyspnea, and cough of an intermittent reversible nature. These symptoms, though, are not unique to asthmatics, and are found in many other respiratory diseases. Some readers are familiar with the term Reactive Airway Disease, an imprecise term used to describe transient symptoms of cough and wheeze when confirmation of a diagnosis of asthma is lacking. The majority of adult patients will already have a diagnosis of asthma since 75% of patients are diagnosed before the age of 7, though asthma can be diagnosed at any age.[18] Therefore, it is not the definition of asthma or necessarily the diagnosis that is important as much as the recognition of the relationship between cough and asthma.

Chronic cough may be the only manifestation of asthma in a condition called cough-variant asthma. Irwin and partners found that, in their prospective study of 102 patients with chronic cough, 28% of asthmatics had only cough as a symptom.[17]

Eosinophilic asthma, distinguished by a high level of eosinophils in the serum, sputum, and tissue, is a particularly severe form of asthma.[19] Though it accounts for only 5% of asthma cases, it is the most common cause of a severe asthma and is most commonly diagnosed in adults between the ages of 35 and 50. Eosinophilic bronchitis is a condition similarly presenting with elevated eosinophils, yet differs in the fact that patients do not exhibit typical variable airway restriction and responsiveness to bronchodilators, which is the defining hallmark of asthma.[20,21] As eosinophilic bronchitis does not respond to bronchoprovocation testing, diagnosis is based on responsiveness to empiric inhaled corticosteroids. It is unclear whether eosinophilic bronchitis is separate from asthma or represents a condition along the spectrum of asthma.[22] Regardless, eosinophilic bronchitis patients invariably present with cough, triggered by inhaled allergens.

Gastroesophageal Reflux and Laryngopharyngeal Reflux

Gastroesophageal reflux disease (GERD) describes the condition where long-term flow of gastric contents flows retrograde from the stomach into the esophagus. Up to 50 episodes of reflux is considered physiologic and, therefore, in order to be classified as GERD, reflux must also cause tissue changes or produce symptoms.[23] Familiarly referred to as heartburn, symptoms of GERD often present with a burning sensation in the chest. It is not uncommon for the pain to be referred to the throat with accompanying globus pharyngeus. More importantly, GERD is a common cause of chronic cough. When refluxate reaches the laryngopharynx (aka both the larynx and hypopharynx), the term laryngopharyngeal reflux (LPR) is used.[24] Unlike GERD, LPR is never considered physiologic.[23]

Reflux is further classified as acidic or nonacidic based upon whether the reflux has a pH less than 4 or greater, respectively. The DeMeester score is an attempt to objectively quantify the results of a pH study and is usually included in results of a reflux study. The DeMeester score is based on calculations from six parameters, including percent total time pH is less than 4, pH less than 4 while in the upright and supine positions, number of reflux episodes, reflux episodes greater than 5 minutes, and the longest reflux episode. A composite score of 14.72 indicates reflux.[25,26] This distinction is important as patients with well-controlled acidic reflux can still have chronic cough in the presence of nonacidic reflux.

The pathophysiologic mechanism by which GERD/LPR causes chronic cough is not well understood, though are several proposed theories.[27] Gastric reflux, in addition to containing hydrochloric acid, also contains proteolytic digestive enzymes, most notably pepsin. Pepsin is formed from its inactive precursor pepsinogen in a process requiring a low pH and, therefore, most efficiently occurs in the stomach. Experiments demonstrate that this conversion of pepsinogen into its active state can occur in a weakly acidic environment up to a pH of 6, a value that would be considered well-treated reflux.[28] Furthermore, pepsin remains in the larynx after a reflux event, and could become activated when a true acidic reflux event occurs. Pepsin may also cause harm through a novel independent mechanism, as proposed by Johnston et al.[29] In Johnston's study, inactivated pepsin is taken in through endocytosis by extraesophageal tissue; once taken into the cell, the pepsin becomes reactivated, leading to mitochondrial and intracellular damage.

Upper Airway Cough Syndrome

Upper airway cough syndrome (UACS) is now the preferred term for the condition previously classified as postnasal drip and is the most common etiology for chronic cough.[30] The latter term is now disfavored, as up to 20% of patients with UACS may not sense and report retrograde flow of mucus into the upper airway.[31] In fact, chronic cough may be the only manifestation of UACS. The transport of sinonasal secretions into the pharynx is a normal physiologic process in heathy individuals, and postnasal drip alone is inadequate to explain the mechanism for chronic cough.

The definition of UACS remains a topic of debate. The American College of Chest Physicians defines UACS as a syndrome characterized by chronic cough related to upper airway abnormalities. As stated above, it is the amalgamation of symptoms including postnasal drip, hence the use of the term syndrome. This difficulty in determining a definition is exacerbated by the fact that there is no objective test to confirm the diagnosis of UACS. Ultimately, it is the response to treatment that defines UACS. Interestingly, postnasal drip is considered by many a symptom rather than a stand-alone condition, and the etiology may be multifactorial, including LPR, allergies, and environmental causes of inflammation with resultant mucus production.[32–34]

Chronic Bronchitis

Chronic bronchitis, along with emphysema, represents a continuum of a condition known as chronic obstructive pulmonary disease (COPD). Emphysema describes a condition where the alveolar walls in the lung weaken and progressively trap air, producing shortness of breath, while chronic bronchitis is defined as the presence of a productive cough lasting at least 3 months for at least 2 consecutive years.[35] Many patients will have features of both chronic bronchitis and emphysema and, therefore, the more encompassing term of COPD is used.

Smoking, either directly or by passive means, is a major risk factor for the development of chronic bronchitis, hence the term "smoker's cough" that is usually associated with this condition.[20] Toxins in cigarette smoke result in inflammation in the lower bronchials. This inflammation then leads to increased mucus production from goblet cells and decreased ciliary function, both of which lead to the distinctive hacking, productive cough.[36] Paradoxically, patients need to be counseled that their cough severity and frequency may worsen temporarily after smoking cessation. Smoking cessation allows cilia to recover their normative function of pulmonary clearance from the lower tracheal bronchial tree into upper airway larynx stimulation cough.

Other Causes of Chronic Cough

Although GERD/LPR, asthma, and upper airway cough syndrome remain the most common causes of chronic cough, clinicians should maintain a broad differential, as there are numerous other pathologies and conditions associated with cough.

In some patients, even after an extensive workup, the etiology of chronic cough cannot be deciphered. Terms used to describe this circumstance include idiopathic, unexplained, refractory, intractable, treatment-resistant, and postviral vagal neuropathic cough.[37] Regardless of the term used, this diagnosis is one of exclusion. More evidence emerges that nonacidic reflux into the proximal esophagus and pharynx that is missed by classic pH-only testing is being discovered on hypopharyngeal-esophageal multichannel intraluminal impedance with dual pH testing and is likely revealing previously missed diagnoses of reflux-induced cough.[38,39]

HISTORY

As a result of the long-standing nature of their symptoms and resulting frustration, it is not uncommon for patients to provide a tangential history, obscuring more relevant details. The history should be focused on the most common causes of chronic cough, maintaining an appreciation for less-frequent sources of chronic cough.

As with any patient assessment, a detailed history and careful physical examination are paramount in the evaluation of chronic cough. The most important information gathered in developing a differential diagnosis for cough is the duration. To review, acute cough is defined by the presence of cough for less than 3 weeks, while chronic cough has a duration of greater than 8 weeks, with subacute cough in between these intervals.

Patients should be queried on inciting triggers of cough. Common triggers include exposure to noxious fumes and perfumes, changes in air temperature, environmental allergens, and posture. Given the numerous etiologies of cough, triggers when pertinent can help to narrow the differential. For example, in a patient with cough exacerbated after eating or laying in the recumbent position, laryngopharyngeal reflux is a more likely diagnosis than asthma.[40,41]

Scrutinizing the family or personal history for atopic disease can favor a diagnosis of allergic rhinitis, asthma, or UACS, given the right clinical context.

Review of Medications

Angiotensin-converting-enzyme (ACE) inhibitors are a class of antihypertensive medication utilized as primary treatment replacing beta-blockers and diuretics. The literature reports an incidence rate of 2% to 33% of chronic cough in those taking ACE inhibitors.[42–44] As such, even when considering the most conservative estimates in prevalence, with the 162 million ACE-inhibitor prescriptions dispensed annually in the United States, the number of patients with chronic cough secondary to ACE inhibitors is substantial.[45] In patients presenting specifically for evaluation of cough, a more recent prospective study cites ACE inhibitors as the etiology in 1% to 3% of cases.[46–48] It is important to note that cough can present at any time while using an ACE inhibitor, even after many years without meaningful cough side effects, and cough is not dose dependent.[49] The only effective means of mitigating ACE-induced cough is complete cessation of medication.[50] ACE inhibitor-induced chronic cough can persist after cessation of therapy and, as such, cannot be excluded as an etiology until a period of weeks has passed.

Social History

Questions regarding alcohol use, recreational drug use—especially those that are inhaled—and tobacco exposure are important when accessing new patients presenting with chronic cough. These questions can be uncomfortable, sensitive, and anxiety provoking for patients and need to be levied in a straightforward, nonjudgmental fashion.

The association between tobacco use and chronic conditions such as lung cancer, emphysema, asthma, heart disease, and, of course, cough is well known. Accordingly, patients should be asked to quantify tobacco use by asking about duration of use, method of delivery, and amount. Patients who smoke are 3 times more likely to develop chronic cough,[51] and multiple studies involving guinea pigs exposed to tobacco smoke have demonstrated increased sensitivity to capsaicin.[52,53] It is also important to be cognizant of passive and environmental tobacco exposure, known more ubiquitously as "secondhand smoke." In a cross-sectional analysis of more than 700 nonsmoking patients, Iribarren et al found that 64% of patients were exposed to at least 9 hours of passive smoke per week, carrying a significant increase in the odds of chronic cough.[54]

A through history necessitates a social history. Tobacco smoke, inhaled either actively or passively, is an obvious interrogation point, but clinicians should also inquire about occupational history as many workers, especially those in industry, are exposed to chemical irritants. Studies estimate 10% of new diagnoses of asthma are the direct result of workplace exposure, highlighting the importance of the occupational history.[55]

PHYSICAL EXAMINATION

Physicians should perform a comprehensive neck examination during the evaluation of a patient with chronic cough. Furthermore, a head and neck examination is not exclusive to an otolaryngologist, nor does it necessitate special equipment. A general examination performed in the office can reveal a supratip crease on the nasal dorsum or venous congestion underneath the eyes, suggestive of allergies. In fact, these physical examination findings are referred to colloquially as the allergic salute and allergic shiners, respectively.

Visualization of the larynx, most commonly performed with a flexible fiberoptic laryngoscope, can reveal signs indicative of GERD/LPR. The Reflux Finding Score is a validated instrument utilized by otolaryngologists to rate the severity of common clinical findings such as subglottic edema, erythema, and excessive mucus.[56] External validation of the RSI affirms good inter- and intrarater reliability though the findings are still subjective and not specific for reflux, but rather serve mainly to support a diagnosis based on history.[57,58] Flexible fiberoptic examination is not only useful in visualizing the effects of GERD/LPR, but many systemic diseases also present with endolaryngeal findings. Sarcoidosis most commonly affects the supraglottic larynx with the vocal cords, also known as the glottis, being the most common site of deposits in amyloidosis. Meanwhile, granulomatosis with polyangitis (Wegener's) deposits are most commonly deposited on the subglottis. One can remember the systemic disease of the larynx with the mnemonic S-A-W, which also conveniently describes the most common location of disease from a cranial caudal direction—sarcoid in the supraglottis, amyloid in the glottis, and Wegener's in the subglottis.

Discussion of the pulmonary physical examination as secondary to the head and neck physical exam may surprise some readers. Admittedly, the emphasis on the head and neck exam can be counterintuitive given cough is physiologically driven by the rapid expulsion of air from the lungs. Findings on lung examination are nonspecific. For instance, an expiratory wheezing can be a sign of asthma, but also presents in COPD, emphysema, or heart failure.

DIAGNOSTIC ADJUNCTS

Imaging

A chest roentgenogram constitutes the most basic diagnostic adjunct to determine cough. Radiographic findings on chest roentgenograms should be addressed expediently, especially when there is concern for malignancy. Low-dose computerized tomography (LDCT) has superior resolution when compared to chest roentgenograms. In a large clinical trial comparing LDCT to chest roentgenograms, LDCT was found to lower mortality in adults between ages 55 and 74 with a 30-pack-per-year history of smoking in fairly good health.[59] However, despite superior resolution, LDCT's utility as a routine screening tool is limited by its high false-positive rate. These incidental false positives subject patients to obligatory invasive workups while incurring additional costs. There remains debate in the literature regarding the optimal screening test for lung cancer, with the American Cancer Society recommending LDCT as a screening tool in select patients, as opposed to chest x-rays, to be performed at centers performing high volumes of LDCT to limit false positive interpretations.[60]

Computerized tomography (CAT) of the paranasal sinus can be used as an adjunct, especially in patients with suspected UACS who previously failed empiric treatments. Pertinent findings on CAT scans include mucosal paranasal sinus thickening and nasal polyposis, strengthening a presumed diagnosis of UACS. CAT scan without contrast is the preferred imaging modality of the paranasal sinuses, as opposed to magnetic resonance imaging, which has a higher false-positive rate than CAT scans. CAT scans should be used judiciously given the healthcare cost and radiation exposure, and guided by history. For example, a CAT scan should not be ordered if the duration of sinonasal symptoms suggests an acute process.[61]

A double pH probe remains the gold standard for diagnosing LPR and should be combined with multichannel impedance testing. Dual probe monitoring demonstrates sensitivity ranging from 50 to 80%. Impedance testing allows for the diagnosis of nonacidic reflux.[62]

Patient Inventories

The Leicester Cough Questionnaire (LCQ) is a validated inventory focused exclusively on health-related quality of life as it pertains to chronic cough.[63] The LCQ consists of 19 items scored on a 7-point Likert scale divided into social, physical, and psychological domains. The inventory is easily self-administered in the outpatient setting, taking less than 5 minutes to complete. An advantage of the LCQ is its repeatability and responsiveness to intervention, making it suitable also to track the progression of treatment efficacy.

The Cough-Specific Quality-of-Life Questionnaire (CQLQ) is another inventory published by the American College of Chest Physicians.[64] The CQLQ, like the LCQ, is a validated self-administered inventory and consists of 28 items scored on a 4-point Likert scale. The CQLQ can be administered to patients with either acute or chronic cough with good reliability and validity.

IMPACT OF COUGH

Bothersome cough is a ubiquitous experience, mainly in the setting of an acute upper respiratory tract infection. Annually, it is estimated that 27 million outpatient clinic visits will be attributed to cough and the most common reason for presentation to primary care.[65] Though extremely prevalent, cough and especially chronic cough remain a challenge for physicians with regard to both diagnosis and treatment. Chronic cough is extremely pervasive, with prevalence estimates ranging from 10% to 20% of the population affected.[66] This is likely an underestimated prevalence given that some patients are unlikely to seek medical treatment, as cough in some patients can either be minimally bothersome or, because of the chronicity of the disease, something patients come to accept as a new normal.[67]

Economic Impact

As stated previously, cough is the most common symptom leading to presentation to primary care physicians. Astonishingly, estimates from an almost 20-year-old report cites almost $250 million spent annually on cough lozenges in the United States—a remarkable figure that is assuredly higher given inflation alone.[68]

A cost breakdown of the typical diagnostic tests and procedures for a patient with chronic cough is shown in Table 1–2. It should be mentioned that the testing listed focuses on the most common causes of cough, and a

Table 1–2. Uninsured Costs of Typical Workup for a Patient with Complex Chronic Cough

Diagnostic Testing	
Chest Roentgenogram	$268.00
Sinus CT Scan	$2,581.00
Modified Barium Swallow	$1,496.00
Procedural Testing	
Allergy Testing	$242.00
pH Impedance Probe	$2,595.00
Spirometry	$537.00
Physician Fee	
Primary Care	
Otolaryngology	
Pulmonology	$2,690.00
Allergy	
Gastroenterology	
Total Cost	$10,409.00

Note. Dollar amounts vary based on location and for this purpose are estimated based on midmajor metropolitan areas with a population of 250,000.[69]

patient with a particularly elusive etiology or who is refractory to typical treatment assuredly would incur more health-care-related costs.

Quality of Life

The study of chronic cough as an academic matter belies the human toll of cough. Chronic cough can be both physically and mentally debilitating and particularly frustrating in those with undetermined cough. Even in those patients whose cough etiology is determined, it is not unusual for the patient to have delayed treatment for months and even years given the multifactorial nature and intrinsic complexities of chronic cough.

In a cross-sectional survey of randomly selected by Ford and associates of more than 4,000 respondents, 12% reported chronic cough. Of these patients, 7% reported cough that either adversely affected activities of daily living (ADL) on at least a weekly basis, with 3% reporting impaired ADLs on a daily basis.[70] Chronic cough when nocturnal can result in significant sleep disruption. Deprivation results in daytime fatigue, malaise, and poor concentration and attention, affecting the patient's professional and personal spheres.

Even in those patients who did not report impaired function, inference from numerous studies would conclude there to be at least a decrease in quality of life. Specifically, physicians need to be aware of depressive symptomatology in the chronic cough patients. Patients can find themselves socially isolated either voluntarily or subconsciously to avoid paroxysm of uncontrolled cough. Activities normally occurring in settings with low ambient noise such as concerts, movies, and church are particularly anxiety provoking. Cough's normal defense mechanism in clearing pathogens and as a response to acute viral illness often causes the false belief that proximity to a patient with chronic cough can in turn result in the transmission of a communicable illnesses. It is not unusual to have patients reporting they are self-conscious in social interactions where friends and coworkers inquire about the patient's cough, often with no malicious intent. Patients with chronic cough can be viewed as overall unhealthy given the numerous related health conditions with chronic cough as a presentation.

Hulme and colleagues investigated the psychological factors associated with cough.[71] In their study, validated inventories accessing for illness perception, anxiety, depression, fatigue, and overall health, among others, were administered to a cross-section of patients treated at a specialty cough referral center and to those without cough. Their investigation found an increase in anxiety, depression, fatigue, and overall somatic symptoms among patients with chronic cough. In their investigation, McGarvey and collaborators specifically studied depression in 100 new patients presenting to a cough specialty center.[72] A validated multi-item questionnaire designed for the assessment of depressive symptomatology was administered to patients at the beginning of enrollment, along with subjective cough scores, and again after 3 months of treatment. At follow-up there was a significant improvement with both subjective cough symptomology and depression indices with the implication of a causal relation between chronic cough and depression.

THINKING OUTSIDE OF THE BOX: CHRONIC COUGH MANAGED THROUGH A MULTIDISCIPLINARY APPROACH

Again, given a significant portion of chronic cough is due to a multifactorial etiology, it should be no surprise that challenging refractory chronic cough too would require an interdisciplinary approach. Given that the most common causes of chronic cough are asthma, GERD/LPR, and UACS, it is logical to value the input of pulmonologist, gastroenterologists, and otolaryngologists or allergists, respectively. There are a limited number of studies that detail the treatment of chronic cough with behavioral management. The studies that are presented would suggest speech-language-pathology-oriented treatments can be helpful, especially those with refractory chronic cough. As such, we advocate for the inclusion of speech-language pathologists among this cadre of specialists. Soni and teammates, in their work with chronic cough patients referred to an academic tertiary laryngology practice, found an incidence of 50% for those who were refractory to comprehensive medical treatment. Of these patients, 85% reported either resolution or near complete resolution of cough symptoms with the inclusion of behavioral management under the auspices of speech-language pathology.[73] On average, patients reported needing two treatment sessions before recognizing improvements and a duration of 6.5 months of treatment for those with complete resolution. In the chronic cough population, where patients are extremely motivated to get better and have a high rapport with their somatic symptoms, improvements from any intervention due to placebo effects need to be considered. In an attempt to address this, Vertigan and fellows reported on their findings from a randomized single-blinded study comparing speech pathology intervention to placebo intervention in patients with chronic cough refractory to medical treatment.[74] The treatment group was educated about the nature of chronic cough, taught suppressive techniques and vocal hygiene, as well as counseled, while patients given placebo treatment were given generalized healthy lifestyle education. While both groups benefited with improving breathing, voicing, and symptom reduction, the group given therapy improved significantly more.

In our tertiary laryngology practice, patients referred for evaluation of chronic cough are seen in conjunction with a speech-language pathologist during their initial visit.

TAKE-HOME POINTS

- Chronic cough is defined as cough persisting for greater than 8 weeks.
- A detailed history and careful physical examination are paramount in the evaluation of chronic cough.
- Assessment of the duration of cough is essential in tailoring a differential diagnosis of cough.
- The most common causes include asthma, GERD/LPR, and upper airway cough syndrome.
- Etiology of cough is often multifactorial.
- Medication lists must be reviewed for the presence of ACE inhibitors, which then need to be discontinued in favor of alternative medications if medically feasible.
- All patients with chronic cough require a chest x-ray at a minimum.
- Cough is the most common reason for presentation to primary care.
- The economic impact associated with the workup of cough is significant and could be individually financially burdensome to the patient.
- Chronic cough can be of great detriment to a patient's quality of life.

REFERENCES

1. Cough. In: *Merriam-Webster.com.* http://www.merriam-webster.com/dictionary/cough. Accessed March 8, 2018.
2. War T. Cause of death for patients with spinal cord injuries. *Arch Intern Med.* 1989;149:1761–1766.
3. Morice A, McGarvey L, Pavord I. Recommendations for the management of cough in adults. *Thorax.* 2006;61(suppl 1), i1–i24.

4. Irwin RS, Baumann MH, Bolser DC, et al. Diagnosis and management of cough executive summary: ACCP evidence-based clinical practice guidelines. *Chest.* 2006;129(suppl 1):1S–23S.
5. Reflex. In: *Merriam-Webster.com.* http://www.merriam-webster.com/dictionary/reflex. Accessed March 8, 2018.
6. Widdicombe J, Fontana G. Cough: what's in a name? *Eur Respir J.* 2006;28(1):10–15.
7. Sharpey-Schafer EP. Effects of coughing on intrathoracic pressure, arterial pressure and peripheral blood flow. *J Physiol.* 1953;122(2):351–357.
8. Comroe J. Special acts involving breathing. *Physiology of Respiration: An Introductory Text.* Chicago, IL: Yearbook Medical Publishers; 1974.
9. Ricco MM, Kummer W, Biglari B, Myers AC, Undem BJ. Interganglionic segregation of distinct vagal afferent fibre phenotypes in guinea-pig airways. *J Physiol.* 1996;496(Pt 2):521–530.
10. Mazzone SB, Canning BJ. Synergistic interactions between airway afferent nerve subtypes mediating reflex bronchospasm in guinea pigs. *Am J Physiol Regul Integr Comp Physiol.* 2002;283(1):R86–R98.
11. Korpás J, Tatár M. The expiration reflex during ontogenesis in the rat. *Physiol Bohemoslov.* 1975;24(3):257–261.
12. Ciba Foundation Symposium. *Breathing: Hering-Breuer Centenary Symposium:* 233.
13. Canning BJ, Chang AB, Bolser DC, et al; CHEST Expert Cough Panel. Anatomy and neurophysiology of cough: Chest Guideline and Expert Panel report. *Chest.* 2014;146(6):1633–1648.
14. Widdicombe JG. Receptors in the trachea and bronchi of the cat. *J Physiol.* 1954;123(1):71–104.
15. Groneberg DA, Niimi A, Dinh QT, et al. Increased expression of transient receptor potential vanilloid-1 in airway nerves of chronic cough. *Am J Respir Crit Care Med.* 2004;170(12):1276–1280.
16. Coleridge JC, Coleridge HM. Afferent vagal C fibre innervation of the lungs and airways and its functional significance. *Rev Physiol Biochem Pharmacol.* 1984;99:1–110.
17. Irwin RS, Boulet LP, Cloutier MM, et al. Managing cough as a defense mechanism and as a symptom: a consensus panel report of the American College of Chest Physicians. *Chest.* 1998;114(2):133S–181S.
18. Yunginger JW, Reed CE, O'Connell EJ, Melton 3rd LJ, O'Fallon WM, Silverstein MD. A community-based study of the epidemiology of asthma. Incidence rates, 1964–1983. *Am Rev Respir Dis.* 1990;146(4):888–894.
19. Bousquet J, Chanez P, Lacoste JV, et al. Eosinophilic inflammation in asthma. *N Engl J Med.* 1990;323(15):1033–1039.
20. Gibson PG, Dolovich J, Denburg J, Ramsdale EH, Hargreave FE. Chronic cough: eosinophilic bronchitis without asthma. *Lancet.* 1989;1(8651):1346–1348.
21. Brightling CE, Ward R, Goh KL, Wardlaw AJ, Pavord ID. Eosinophilic bronchitis is an important cause of chronic cough. *Am J Respir Crit Care Med.* 1999;160(2):406–410.
22. Brightling CE, Symon FA, Birring SS, Bradding P, Wardlaw AJ, Pavord ID. Comparison of airway immunopathology of eosinophilic bronchitis and asthma. *Thorax.* 2003;58(6):528–532.

23. Koufman JA. The otolaryngologic manifestations of gastroesophageal reflux disease (GERD): a clinical investigation of 225 patients using ambulatory 24-hour pH monitoring and an experimental investigation of the role of acid and pepsin in the development of laryngeal injury. *Laryngoscope,* 1991;101(S53):1–78.
24. Koufman JA, Aviv JE, Casiano RR, Shaw GY. Laryngopharyngeal reflux: position statement of the committee on speech, voice, and swallowing disorders of the American Academy of Otolaryngology-Head and Neck Surgery. *Otolaryngol Head Neck Surg.* 2002;127(1):32–35.
25. Johnson, LF, Demeester TR. Twenty-four-hour pH monitoring of the distal esophagus. *Am J Gastroenterol,* 1974;62(4):325–332.
26. DeMeester TR, Wang CI, Wernly JA, et al. Technique, indications, and clinical use of 24 hour esophageal pH monitoring. *J Thorac Cardiovasc Surg.* 1980;79(5): 656–670.
27. Barry DW, Vaezi MF. Laryngopharyngeal reflux: more questions than answers. *Cleve Clin J Med.* 2010;77(5):327–334.
28. Ludemann JP, Manoukian J, Shaw K, Bernard C, Davis M, al-Jubab A. Effects of simulated gastroesophageal reflux on the untraumatized rabbit larynx. *J Otolaryngol.* 1998;27(3):127–131.
29. Johnston N, Yan JC, Hoekzema CR, et al. Pepsin promotes proliferation of laryngeal and pharyngeal epithelial cells. *Laryngoscope.* 2012;122(6):1317–1325.
30. Pratter MR. Chronic upper airway cough syndrome secondary to rhinosinus diseases (previously referred to as postnasal drip syndrome): ACCP evidence-based clinical practice guidelines. *Chest.* 2006;129(suppl 1):63S–71S.
31. Pratter MR, Bartter T, Akers S, DuBois J. An algorithmic approach to chronic cough. *Ann Intern Med.* 1993;119(10):977–983.
32. Morice AH. Post-nasal drip syndrome—a symptom to be sniffed at? *Pulm Pharmacol Ther.* 2004;17(6):343–345.
33. O'Hara J, Jones N. "Post-nasal drip syndrome": most patients with purulent nasal secretions do not complain of chronic cough. *Rhinology.* 2006;44(4):270–273.
34. Sanu A, Eccles R. Postnasal drip syndrome. Two hundred years of controversy between UK and USA. *Rhinology.* 2008;46(2):86.
35. Kim V, Criner GJ. Chronic bronchitis and chronic obstructive pulmonary disease. *Am J Respir Crit Care Med.* 2013;187(3):228–237.
36. Hogg JC. Pathophysiology of airflow limitation in chronic obstructive pulmonary disease. *Lancet.* 2004;364(9435);709–721.
37. Gibson P, Wang G, McGarvey L, Vertigan AE, Altman KW, Birring SS. Treatment of unexplained chronic cough: chest guideline and expert panel report. *Chest.* 2016;149(1):27–44.
38. Hoppo T, Komatsu Y, Jobe BA. Antireflux surgery in patients with chronic cough and abnormal proximal exposure as measured by hypopharyngeal multichannel intraluminal impedance. *JAMA Surgery.* 2013;148(7):608–605.
39. Zerbib F, Roman S, Ropert A, et al. Esophageal pH-impedance monitoring and symptom analysis in GERD: a study in patients off and on therapy. *Am J Gastroenterol.* 2006;101(9):1956.
40. Hamilton JW, Boisen RJ Yamamoto DT, Wagner JL, Reichelderfer M. Sleeping on a wedge diminishes exposure of the esophagus to refluxed acid. *Dig Dis Sci.* 1988;33(5);518–522.

41. Khoury RM, Camacho-Lobato L, Katz PO, Mohiuddin MA, Castell DO. Influence of spontaneous sleep positions on nighttime recumbent reflux in patients with gastroesophageal reflux disease. *Am J Gastroenterol.* 1999;94(8):2069.
42. Fox AJ, Lalloo UG, Belvisi MG, Bernareggi M, Chung KF, Barnes PJ. Bradykinin–evoked sensitization of airway sensory nerves: a mechanism for ACE–inhibitor cough. *Nat Med.* 1996;2(7):814.
43. Choudry NB, Fuller RW, Pride NB. Sensitivity of the human cough reflex: effect of inflammatory mediators prostaglandin E2, bradykinin, and histamine. *Am Rev Respir Dis.* 1989;140(1):137–141.
44. Nichol G, Nix A, Barnes PJ, Chung KF. Prostaglandin F2 alpha enhancement of capsaicin induced cough in man: modulation by beta-2 adrenergic and anticholinergic drugs. *Thorax.* 1990;45(9):694–698.
45. Health I. Top therapeutic classes by U.S. dispensed prescriptions. http://www.imshealth.com/deployedfiles/imshealth/%20U.S.RXs.pdf. Published 2016. Accessed March 11, 2018
46. Irwin RS, Curley FJ, French CL. Chronic cough. The spectrum and frequency of causes, key components of the diagnostic evaluation, and outcome of specific therapy. *Am Rev Respir Dis.* 1990;141(3):640–647.
47. Smyrnios NA, Irwin RS, Curley FJ. Chronic cough with a history of excessive sputum production: the spectrum and frequency of causes, key components of the diagnostic evaluation, and outcome of specific therapy. *Chest.* 1995;108(4):991–997.
48. Mello CJ, Irwin RS, Curley FJ. Predictive values of the character, timing, and complications of chronic cough in diagnosing its cause. *Arch Intern Med.* 1996;156(9):997–1003.
49. Israili ZH, Hall WD. Cough and angioneurotic edema associated with angiotensin-converting enzyme inhibitor therapy: a review of the literature and pathophysiology. *Ann Intern Med.* 1992;117(3):234–242.
50. Dicpinigaitis PV. Angiotensin-converting enzyme inhibitor-induced cough: ACCP evidence-based clinical practice guidelines. *Chest.* 2006;129(1):169S–173S.
51. Zemp E, Elsasser S, Schindler C, et al. Long-term ambient air pollution and respiratory symptoms in adults (SAPALDIA study). The SAPALDIA Team. *Am J Respir Crit Care Med.* 1999;159(4 pt 1):1257–1266.
52. Lewis CA, Ambrose C, Banner K, et al. Animal models of cough: literature review and presentation of a novel cigarette smoke-enhanced cough model in the guinea-pig. *Pulm Pharmacol Ther.* 2007;20(4):325–333.
53. Bergren DR. Chronic tobacco smoke exposure increases cough to capsaicin in awake guinea pigs. *Respir Physiol.* 2001;126(2):127–140.
54. Iribarren C, Friedman GD, Klatsky AL, Eisner MD. Exposure to environmental tobacco smoke: association with personal characteristics and self reported health conditions. *J Epidemiol Community Health.* 2001;55(10):721–728.
55. Kogevinas M, Zock JP, Jarvis D, et al. Exposure to substances in the workplace and new-onset asthma: an international prospective population-based study (ECRHS-II). *Lancet.* 2007;370(9584):336–341.
56. Belafsky, PC, Postma GN, Koufman JA. The validity and reliability of the reflux finding score (RFS). *Laryngoscope.* 2001;111(8):1313–1317.
57. Ivey CM, Welge J, Steward DL. Validation of the reflux finding score (RFS) for chronic laryngopharyngitis. *Otolaryngol Head Neck Surg.* 2004;131(2):P131.

58. Branski RC, Bhattacharyya, N, Shapiro J. The reliability of the assessment of endoscopic laryngeal findings associated with laryngopharyngeal reflux disease. *Laryngoscope.* 2002;112(6):1019–1024.
59. Team NLSTR. The national lung screening trial: overview and study design. *Radiology.* 2011;258(1):243–253.
60. Wender R, Fontham ET, Barrera Jr E, et al. American Cancer Society lung cancer screening guidelines. *CA Cancer J Clin.* 2013;63(2):106–117.
61. Rosenfeld RM, Piccirillo JF, Chandrasekhar SS, et al. Clinical practice guideline (update): adult sinusitis. *Otolaryngol Head Neck Surg.* 2015;152(suppl 2);S1–S39.
62. Postma GN. Ambulatory pH monitoring methodology. *Ann Otol Rhinol Laryngol Suppl.* 2000;184;10–14.
63. Birring SS, Prudon B, Carr AJ, Singh SJ, Morgan MD, Pavord ID. Development of a symptom specific health status measure for patients with chronic cough: Leicester Cough Questionnaire (LCQ). *Thorax.* 2003;58(4):339–343.
64. French CT, Irwin RS, Fletcher KE, Adams TM. Evaluation of a cough-specific quality-of-life questionnaire. *Chest.* 2002;121(4):1123–1131.
65. Woodwell D. National ambulatory medical care survey: 1998 outpatient department summary. *Adv Data.* 2000;317:1–23.
66. Barbee RA, Halonen M, Kaltenborn WT, Burrows B. A longitudinal study of respiratory symptoms in a community population sample. Correlations with smoking, allergen skin-test reactivity, and serum IgE. *Chest.* 1991;99(1):20–26.
67. Chung KF, Pavord ID. Prevalence, pathogenesis, and causes of chronic cough. *Lancet.* 2008;371(9621):1364–1374.
68. Kauffmann F, Varraso R. The epidemiology of cough. *Pulm Pharmacol Ther.* 2011;24(3):289–294.
69. Health, F. Estimate Health Care Expenses 2017. http://www.fairhealthconsumer.org. Accessed March 11, 2018.
70. Ford AC, Forman D, Moayyedi P, Morice AH. Cough in the community: a cross sectional survey and the relationship to gastrointestinal symptoms. *Thorax.* 2006;61(11):975–979.
71. Hulme K, Deary V, Dogan S, Parker SM. Psychological profile of individuals presenting with chronic cough. *ERJ Open Res.* 2017;3(1):00099–2016.
72. McGarvey LP, Carton C, Gamble LA, et al. Prevalence of psychomorbidity among patients with chronic cough. *Cough.* 2006;2:4.
73. Soni RS, Ebersole B, Jamal N. Treatment of chronic cough: Single-institution experience utilizing behavioral therapy. *Otolaryngol Head Neck Surg.* 2017;156(1):103–108.
74. Vertigan AE, Theodoros DG, Gibson PG, Winkworth AL. Efficacy of speech pathology management for chronic cough: a randomised placebo controlled trial of treatment efficacy. *Thorax.* 2006;61(12):1065–1069.

2

COUGH-VARIANT ASTHMA AND RELATED DISEASES

Nicole L. Grossman and Christopher H. Fanta

INTRODUCTION

Asthma is one of the most common causes of chronic cough, accounting for 24% to 29% of cases of chronic cough in nonsmoking individuals.[1–3] Asthma usually manifests as some combination of cough, wheeze, shortness of breath, and chest tightness. A subgroup of asthmatic patients, however, report cough as their main—and sometimes even only—symptom.[4] These individuals are described as having cough-variant asthma. On its own, cough-variant asthma accounts for about 30% of referrals to cough clinics.[5,6] This chapter will focus on the diagnosis and treatment of asthma, with special attention given to the cough-variant asthma phenotype.

PATHOPHYSIOLOGY

The term "asthma" originates from the Greek root ασθμαινω, meaning "to pant heavily" or "to gasp for breath."[7] Over time, the term has evolved to describe a heterogeneous inflammatory disease characterized pathologically by airway wall inflammation, areas of airway epithelial desquamation, subepithelial collagen deposition, goblet cell hyperplasia with mucous hypersecretion, and smooth muscle hypertrophy and hyperplasia; and physiologically by variable airflow obstruction and persistent bronchial hyperresponsiveness. Along the asthma disease spectrum are many subgroups (or phenotypes), including atopic asthma, neutrophilic asthma, exercise-induced bronchoconstriction (EIB), obese asthma, the asthma-chronic obstructive pulmonary disease overlap syndrome (ACOS), occupational asthma, aspirin-exacerbated respiratory disease (AERD), exacerbation-prone asthma, and cough-variant asthma, to name a few. While each of these asthma phenotypes has its unique pathobiology, they all share the backbone-defining feature of asthma—variable expiratory airflow limitation (and the consequent symptoms of cough, wheeze, shortness of breath, and/or chest tightness that vary over time and in intensity).

Acute airway obstruction in asthma is driven by a combination of airway smooth muscle constriction and bronchial inflammation. Airway narrowing and the mediators released as part of airway inflammation in asthma trigger the cough receptors that line the airways, stimulating the cough reflex. Bronchoconstriction can occur in response to many different environmental stimuli, including inhaled allergens, irritants, respiratory infections, cold air, and certain medications such as beta blockers. Asthmatic patients appear to have a unique infiltration of their airway smooth muscle cells by activated mast cells,[8,9] resulting in increased airway smooth muscle mass and airway hyperresponsiveness. Allergen-induced airway narrowing, one of the more common causes of bronchoconstriction, results predominantly from IgE-dependent release of the mast cell-derived mediators, including histamine, tryptase, leukotrienes, and prostaglandins.[10] These mast cell mediators directly contract airway smooth muscle cells and promote airway infiltration with inflammatory cells, especially eosinophils.

Airway inflammation in asthma results from activation of mast cells and T helper 1 (Th1) and T helper 2 (Th2) lymphocytes. Th2 cell activation leads to the release of the cytokines interleukin-4 (IL-4), IL-5, and IL-13, which in turn leads to increased bone marrow release of eosinophils. Airway eosinophilia is a major contributor to the inflammatory cycle of asthma. There is developing evidence that airway and sputum neutrophilia also contribute to a corticosteroid-resistant asthma phenotype in some patients.

With persistent airway inflammation, individuals with asthma develop mucous hypersecretion, mucous plugging of the airways, and mucosal, submucosal, and adventitial edema. Mucous plugging, airway edema, subepithelial fibrosis, smooth muscle hypertrophy, and smooth muscle hyperplasia can result in permanent structural changes in the airways, referred to as remodeling. Remodeled airways can become permanently obstructed, rendering them less responsive to traditional therapy, with features akin to chronic obstructive pulmonary disease (COPD).

Interestingly, the mechanism of cough in asthma has features that are likely somewhat distinct from the above-mentioned pathways that induce bronchial hyperresponsiveness. Individuals with cough-variant asthma have a hypersensitive cough reflex but demonstrate less bronchial hyperresponsiveness to methacholine than those with classic asthma.[11,12]

CLINICAL MANIFESTATIONS

Of the approximately 26 million Americans with asthma (8.4% of the population), more than 75% of cases first manifest in childhood as cough, wheeze, chest tightness, or frequent chest colds.[13] Persistent cough is a frequent manifestation of childhood asthma. Patients with asthma may experience a period of disease latency during their teenage years. Some then outgrow their disease, and others have a resurgence of symptoms. Poor, female, Black, and Puerto Rican individuals are disproportionately affected by asthma.[14] This is likely due to a combination of genetic, environmental, and socioeconomic factors.

The typical manifestations of asthma include any combination of cough, wheeze, chest tightness, or shortness of breath that varies over time and in intensity, and improves with bronchodilators. Because of the variable nature of bronchospasm, individuals with asthma can lack airflow obstruction and be asymptomatic (including cough-free) when evaluated in a care provider's office. A thorough history, however, should reveal fluctuating symptoms that result from usual triggers. These triggers commonly include upper respiratory tract infections, exercise, environmental allergens (including dust mites, seasonal pollens, animal dander, cockroaches, mice, molds, and work-related allergic exposures), strong emotions, cold air, cigarette smoke, and strong odors or fumes. A small percentage of adults with asthma will develop asthmatic symptoms after ingestion of aspirin or any nonsteroidal anti-inflammatory drug. They often have associated nasal symptoms and/or nasal polyps, leading to the encompassing descriptor, aspirin-exacerbated respiratory disease.

While many patients present with the classic combination of triggered cough, wheeze, chest tightness, and shortness of breath, there exists a subgroup of previously mentioned individuals with asthma who have cough-variant (or cough-predominant) asthma. These individuals frequently lack wheeze, chest tightness, and dyspnea but have heightened cough reflex sensitivity with dry or minimally productive cough. Longitudinal studies suggest that nearly 33% of patients with cough-variant asthma will develop the classical symptom of asthmatic wheeze over time.[15,16]

DIAGNOSIS

The diagnosis of asthma is made by clinical history consistent with asthma, exclusion of alternate diagnoses, demonstration of variable airflow obstruction on spirometry, and resolution of symptoms with antiasthmatic therapy. Episodic cough, wheeze, and shortness of breath can be caused by many diseases, so it is critical to disentangle asthma signs and symptoms from those of mimicking and comorbid disorders, from the common (such as recurrent chest infections, gastroesophageal reflux, chronic rhinosinusitis, and seasonal allergies) to the uncommon (such as paradoxical vocal fold motion disorder, eosinophilic granulomatosis with polyangiitis, acute or chronic eosinophilic pneumonia, allergic bronchopulmonary aspergillosis, hypersensitivity pneumonitis, and infections with associated eosinophilia, like strongyloidiasis and filariasis). This section will focus on the diagnostic modalities used to distinguish asthma from other disorders.

Spirometry

Spirometry is the most widely used pulmonary function test that enables the clinician to evaluate for obstructive lung disease. Patients are coached to inhale maximally and then quickly and forcefully exhale their complete breath into a spirometer. The spirometer measures the forced expiratory volume in the first second (FEV_1) and total forced expired volume, or forced vital capacity (FVC). These values are used to calculate an FEV_1/FVC ratio. Airflow obstruction has generally been defined as an FEV_1/FVC ratio less than 0.7. More accurately (because it takes into account changes in FEV_1/FVC with age), airflow obstruction is defined as a value less than the lower limit of normal, the fifth percentile of the spirometer's electronically computed 95% confidence intervals. If airflow obstruction is present, the severity of obstruction is then determined by the percent predicted reduction in FEV_1. For example, if the FEV_1 is 3 L (75% of predicted) and the FVC is 5 L (95% of predicted), the FEV_1/FVC ratio of 0.6 demonstrates the presence of airflow obstruction and the FEV_1 at 75% of predicted is used to describe the severity of airflow obstruction as mild.

Airflow obstruction can also be identified with a classic scooped, concave shape on the expiratory limb of a flow-volume loop (Figure 2–1). As the name implies, flow-volume loops are a graphic representation of expiratory (and inspiratory) air volume versus rate of airflow.

Bronchodilator Reversibility and Bronchoprovocation Testing

Variability in measured airflow obstruction is essential to asthma diagnosis. Variability can be seen over time or in response to bronchodilator or bronchoprovocation testing.[17]

If a patient has verified obstruction on his or her spirometry (with FEV_1/FVC less than 0.7), a diagnosis of variable airflow obstruction can be made by demonstrating significant FEV_1 improvement on subsequent testing performed longitudinally or immediately following bronchodilator administration. Bronchodilator reversibility testing is performed by

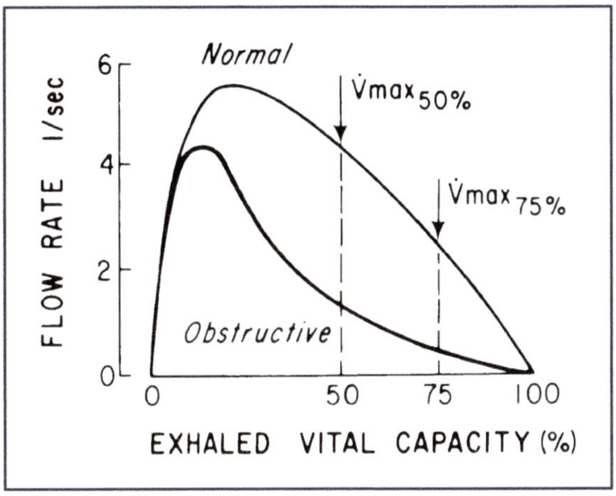

Figure 2–1. Expiratory flow-volume curve. A maximal forced exhalation is displayed as flow (vertical axis) as a function of exhaled volume (horizontal axis). The thin black line gives the normal predicted values; the thick black line illustrates the expiratory flow-volume curve seen in persons with obstructive lung diseases, such as asthma. Maximal expiratory flow at 50% and at 75% of the exhaled vital capacity are shown as $Vmax_{50\%}$ and $Vmax_{75\%}$, respectively.

administering two to four puffs (or a nebulized treatment) of a short-acting bronchodilator after initial spirometry, and repeating the spirometry 10 to 15 minutes later. If a patient's FEV_1 increases by 12% with an absolute change of 200 cc, he or she is said to have a positive response to bronchodilator. There is no clearly defined bronchodilator reversibility cutoff for asthma diagnosis, though some providers look for a 15% or 20% increase in FEV_1 after administration of bronchodilator. There are rare circumstances when a patient with asthma might have a false negative response (less than 12% or less than 200 cc improvement) to bronchodilator testing. The potential causes for failure of lung function to improve following bronchodilator administration in asthma are beyond the scope of this chapter.

If a patient does not have obstruction on his or her spirometry (with FEV_1/FVC greater than 0.7), but a diagnosis of asthma is still suspected, bronchoprovocation testing can be performed to induce bronchoconstriction. Patients with asthma are more sensitive than normal to provocative airway stimuli and, therefore, in response to these stimuli, experience airflow obstruction with a significant decrease in FEV_1. A variety of bronchoprovocative agents can be used, including methacholine, mannitol, exercise, and eucapnic hyperventilation of cold, dry air. Methacholine challenge is considered the gold standard and involves inhalation of incrementally increasing concentrations of methacholine, an analog of the neurotransmitter acetylcholine, with spirometry testing after each inhalation (Figure 2–2). The test concludes when the subject experiences a 20% relative reduction in FEV_1 or reaches the maximum concentration of inhaled methacholine. The methacholine concentration at which a 20% reduction is seen is called the provocative concentration, or PC_{20}. A PC_{20} greater than 16 mg/mL excludes an asthma diagnosis with reasonable certainty; a PC_{20} less than 8 mg/mL indicates bronchial hyperresponsiveness consistent with asthma. The test lacks specificity, unfortunately, as more than 5% of the general population without asthma may also have a significant decrease in FEV_1 in response to methacholine (false positives).

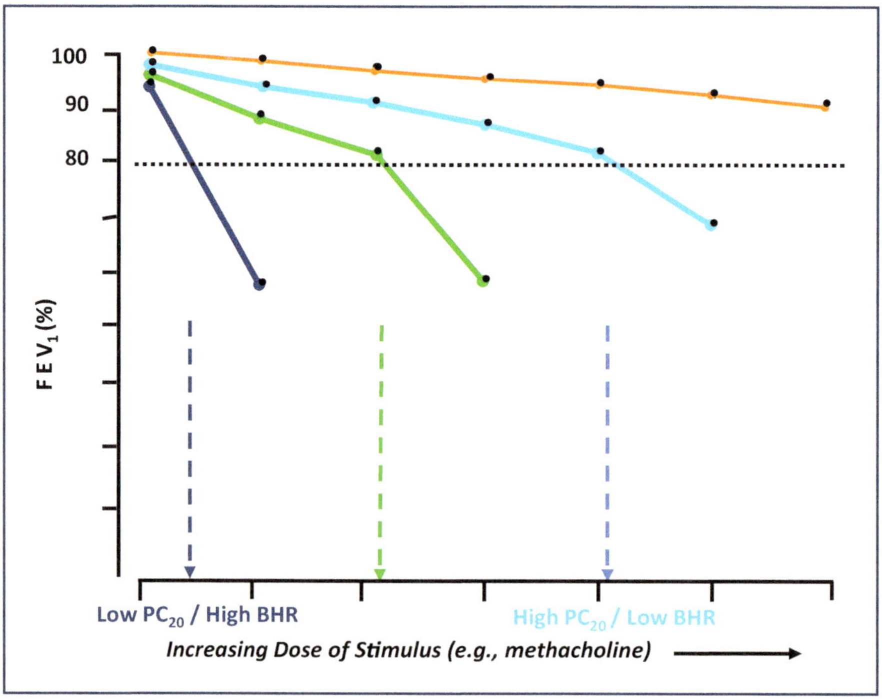

Figure 2–2. Schematic representation of bronchoprovocation challenges in four subjects. The response (in terms of change in FEV_1 as a percent of baseline) to increasing doses of a bronchoprovocative stimulus such as methacholine is shown for one subject without bronchial hyperresponsiveness (orange curve) and 3 subjects exhibiting differing degrees of bronchial hyperresponsiveness. The most responsive (with the lowest PC_{20}) is shown in dark blue; the least responsive (with the highest PC_{20}) is shown in pale blue. BHR = bronchial hyperresponsiveness; PC_{20} = the provocative concentration of methacholine causing a 20% fall from baseline in FEV_1. The dashed vertical lines mark extrapolation along the curves to the dose of methacholine causing a 20% fall in FEV_1 from baseline. (Note: the initial FEV_1 in all subjects is set at 100%; the dots indicating initial FEV_1 are separated only for clarity of the image.)

Serum Biomarkers and Fractional Exhaled Nitric Oxide

A diagnostic serum or exhaled breath biomarker specific for asthma or asthma-induced cough has yet to be discovered. In Th2-driven asthma, patients may have increased peripheral eosinophils and IgE, in addition to increased airway mucosal eosinophilia. Airway mucosal eosinophilia is not limited to asthma, however; it is found in other Th2-driven airway diseases as well, like eosinophilic bronchitis and, in some patients, COPD. Mucosal eosinophilia can be approximated by measuring sputum eosinophils. Traditionally, sputum eosinophils greater than or equal to 2% to 3% of the total sputum white cell count indicate Th2 airway inflammation. However, induced sputum eosinophils are not measured in routine practice because we lack consistent standards of sputum induction, processing, and interpretation. Fractional exhaled nitric oxide (F_{ENO}), a noninvasive surrogate of mucosal eosinophilia, is used more routinely. Fractional exhaled nitric oxide correlates well with induced sputum eosinophils, presumably because eosinophilic airway inflammation leads to upregulation of inducible nitric oxide synthase in respiratory epithelial cells with release of nitric oxide into the exhaled breath. In a recent meta-analysis, F_{ENO} was shown to have 66% sensitivity and 76% specificity in detecting ≥3% induced sputum eosinophils.[18] $F_{ENO} > 47$ ppb predicts corticosteroid responsiveness with a negative predictive value of 89%. In one study, elevated F_{ENO} correlated with corticosteroid responsiveness better than spirometry, bronchodilator response, variation in peak flow, or methacholine airway hyperresponsiveness.[19]

In summary, objective testing is available to rule in or rule out a diagnosis of asthma. A person with normal lung function and no evidence of airflow obstruction at a time when he or she is actively coughing almost certainly does not have asthma as the cause of cough. Similarly, a negative bronchoprovocation challenge excludes asthma as the cause of cough with at least 95% certainty. On the other hand, a person with cough and reversible airflow obstruction can be assumed to have asthma as at least one potential cause of coughing and should be treated for asthma until normal (or optimal) lung function is achieved. In general, asthma is exquisitely sensitive to treatment with corticosteroids. Cough that is not ameliorated by a course of oral corticosteroids (eg, prednisone 40 mg/day for 1–2 weeks) is probably not due to asthma. At the same time, making a diagnosis of asthma based solely on clinical impression, without confirmation based on objective (spirometric) testing, is fraught with potential for error. In a recent study of 467 adults with a physician's diagnosis of asthma made within the previous 5 years, a full 33% were found not to have current asthma on detailed medical review and pulmonary function testing. More than half of the patients with an erroneous diagnosis of asthma had not had pulmonary function testing at the time of diagnosis.[20]

TREATMENT

Patients with classic asthma and cough-variant asthma are treated similarly. The pillars to achieving asthma control are trigger avoidance, patient self-awareness and monitoring of symptoms, strong patient-physician communication, and medication compliance with correct inhaler technique and appropriate medications.[21] Asthma therapy should be initiated once reversible airway obstruction has been confirmed in a patient with classic asthma symptoms or chronic cough. We understand that under certain circumstances, it may be desirable to begin an empiric trial of therapy for suspected asthma in a patient with chronic cough based on history and examination alone. However, in this circumstance when reversible airway obstruction has not been confirmed, a symptomatic response to steroid therapy cannot exclude other etiologies of steroid-responsive cough and therefore does not establish a diagnosis of asthma.

Asthma medications are divided into two classes: quick-relief bronchodilators and controller medications. These are both described in detail below.

Quick-Relief Bronchodilators

All patients with asthma, including those with mild disease, should have access to quick-relief inhalers. Inhaled short-acting beta-adrenergic agonists (referred to as short-acting beta-agonists, or SABAs) induce bronchodilation of constricted airways in less than 5 minutes. In instances of acute bronchoconstriction, SABAs therefore quickly reverse airflow obstruction and relieve debilitating symptoms of cough, wheeze, shortness of breath, and chest tightness.

Albuterol is the most commonly used short-acting bronchodilator. Its peak effect occurs 30 to 60 minutes after inhalation, and its duration of efficacy is about 4 to 6 hours.[22] Patients should be instructed to take two puffs of their quick-relief inhaler at the onset of asthma symptoms, or proactively 20 to 30 minutes before an exposure to known symptom triggers to prevent bronchoconstriction.

Albuterol is a racemic mixture of dextro- and levostereoisomers. Levalbuterol is a single-isomer preparation developed with the hope of reducing the adverse stimulatory side effects of albuterol. However, most studies have found the activity and side-effect profiles of albuterol and levalbuterol to be indistinguishable.

Asthma outcomes do not improve when short-acting bronchodilators are used regularly, 4 times daily, compared to on an as-needed basis.[23] A disadvantage to regular use of SABAs is the development of tolerance, or tachyphylaxis, to their bronchoprotective effect. After regular use for as little as 1 week, the ability of albuterol to protect against exercise-induced bronchoconstriction when taken prior to exercise diminishes significantly. Once a patient is using his or her SABA more than twice per week to relieve daytime asthma symptoms or more than twice per month to relieve nocturnal symptoms, consensus is to step up therapy by adding a long-acting controller medication.

Controller Agents

Refer to Table 2–1. Long-term asthma management is approached in a stepwise fashion, with medication adjustments dependent upon symptom control and exacerbation frequency. Medication regimens should be escalated (or stepped up) until adequate disease control is achieved. Conversely,

Table 2–1. Controller Medications Available to Treat Asthma

Medication	Trade Name	Formulation
Inhaled corticosteroids		
Beclomethasone	*Qvar*	DPI
Budesonide	*Pulmicort*	DPI, liquid for nebulization
Ciclesonide	*Alvesco*	MDI
Flunisolide	*Aerospan*	MDI
Fluticasone furoate	*Arnuity*	DPI
Fluticasone propionate	*Armonair; Flovent*	DPI; MDI and DPI
Mometasone	*Asmanex*	MDI and DPI
Leukotriene modifiers		
Montelukast	*Singulair*	Tablet
Zafirlukast	*Accolate*	Tablet
Zileuton	*Zyflo*	Tablet
Long-acting beta-agonist bronchodilators with inhaled corticosteroids		
Formoterol + budesonide	*Symbicort*	MDI
Formoterol + mometasone	*Dulera*	MDI
Salmeterol + fluticasone propionate	*Advair; AirDuo*	MDI and DPI; DPI
Vilanterol + fluticasone furoate	*Breo*	DPI

Note. DPI = dry-powder inhaler; MDI = metered-dose inhaler.

patients with excellent clinical control should have their regimens evaluated for deintensification (or stepping down) to avoid excess steroid exposure.

The escalation ladder of asthma controller therapy starts with inhaled corticosteroids (ICS), followed by the addition of long-acting beta agonists (LABAs), leukotriene modifiers, biologic therapies, and oral steroids. Other therapies used in some cases to improve asthma control and reduce exacerbations include long-acting muscarinic antagonists,[24] macrolide antibiotics,[25] and bronchial thermoplasty.[26]

Inhaled Corticosteroids

Inhaled corticosteroids are the mainstay of long-term asthma control. They are the first controller medication that should be added to a patient's regimen if his or her disease is not well controlled with SABAs alone. Inhaled corticosteroids suppress asthma-related cough and are associated with fewer asthma symptoms, improved lung function, improved asthma-specific quality of life, and fewer asthma exacerbations. They reduce the risk of severe exacerbations and asthma-related deaths.[27] Inhaled corticosteroids can even be used to abort mild to moderate asthma exacerbations by quadrupling the regular dose at the onset of worsening asthma symptoms.[28]

Inhaled corticosteroids are thought to work by decreasing inflammatory activity in the airway mucosa and submucosa. Specifically, they suppress mast cell, eosinophil, T- lymphocyte, and dendritic cell activation.[29] As a result, they decrease F_{ENO} and sputum eosinophils, and these biomarkers can be used not only as indicators of corticosteroid responsiveness, but also as markers of compliance with steroid use. Inhaled steroids also significantly reduce goblet cell hyperplasia and bronchial hyperresponsiveness.[30,31]

It is important to note that inhaled corticosteroids do not cure individuals of asthma; they only suppress the aforementioned inflammatory activity and subsequent bronchial hyperresponsiveness. Within about 2 weeks of inhaled corticosteroid cessation, F_{ENO}, sputum eosinophils, and bronchial hyperresponsiveness have been observed to return to baseline.[32,33]

Few systemic side effects are observed at low to medium doses of inhaled corticosteroids. Patients can develop sore throat, cough with medication delivery, dysphonia, and pharyngeal or laryngeal candidiasis. These side effects can be minimized by using a spacer delivery device ("valved holding chamber") and by rinsing the mouth after each use. Long-term use of inhaled corticosteroids in high doses (defined as ≥1000 μg of beclomethasone, or the equivalent, per day) can cause accelerated loss of bone mass, elevated intraocular pressure, development of cataracts, and increased bruising. These side effect risks are still significantly less frequent and less severe than those associated with long-term use of systemic corticosteroids. Therefore, high-dose inhaled corticosteroids are often used to treat patients with severe persistent asthma. Inhaled steroids in children are associated with slightly impaired growth rates, with loss on average of approximately 1 cm of predicted adult height.

While high-dose inhaled steroids are clinically used to control severe asthma, clinicians must be cognizant of the therapeutic ceiling effect of inhaled corticosteroids. Using bronchial hyperresponsiveness (PC20) as the readout, there is little additional benefit from incremental doses of inhaled steroids above approximately 670 μg/day of beclomethasone or the equivalent; the dose-response curve is flat. Unfortunately, the systemic absorption curve is relatively linear. Thus, at a patient-specific dose of inhaled corticosteroid, the adverse systemic effects of increasing inhaled corticosteroids may outpace the therapeutic benefits.

Long-Acting Beta Agonists

We add long-acting beta agonists (LABAs) to an individual's asthma regimen when his or her disease is uncontrolled with inhaled corticosteroid monotherapy. LABAs should not be used in isolation without an inhaled corticosteroid. When used in conjunction with inhaled corticosteroids, they reduce nighttime and daytime symptoms, improve lung function, lower exacerbation risk, and reduce the dose of inhaled corticosteroid needed to maintain control of symptoms.

In late 2017, the black box warning on asthma management with LABAs in conjunction with inhaled corticosteroids was lifted. While the Salmeterol Multicenter Asthma Research Trial (SMART) had previously found an increased mortality among individuals randomized to salmeterol plus usual therapy (versus placebo plus usual therapy),[34] four subsequent large clinical safety trials demonstrated that combination therapy with LABAs and inhaled corticosteroids does not increase mortality and in fact reduces asthma exacerbations compared to treatment with inhaled corticosteroids alone.[35,36]

Leukotriene Modifiers

Leukotriene receptor antagonists are occasionally used in mild persistent asthma as the initial controller agent, in place of inhaled corticosteroids. They are conveniently administered as a tablet taken once or twice daily and have rare side effects (specifically, mood alteration and depression). In addition, they can be added to inhaled corticosteroid regimens when asthma is severe. A small, randomized, placebo-controlled trial in patients with cough-variant asthma suggested that the leukotriene receptor antagonist zafirlukast improved subjective cough scores and cough-reflex sensitivity. Additionally, people with asthma who smoke,[37] are obese,[38] or have aspirin-exacerbated respiratory disease[39] may derive particular benefit from leukotriene modifiers. Ultimately, however, it is believed that inhaled corticosteroids and combination ICS/LABA therapy are more effective in treating classic asthma than the leukotriene receptor antagonists.

Biologic Therapy

Despite the use of short-acting beta agonists, inhaled corticosteroids, LABAs, and leukotriene receptor antagonists, about 10 to 20% of patients with asthma continue to have debilitating symptoms and frequent exacerbations. Fortunately, research into targeted therapies in asthma has expanded significantly over the last decade, with a particular focus on biologic, phenotype-targeted therapies. A number of monoclonal antibody therapies have emerged that significantly reduce asthma exacerbations and improve asthma symptoms in an otherwise difficult-to-control disease.

Currently, there are 5 FDA-approved biologic therapies. They target Th2-driven atopic asthma by blocking IgE or inhibiting IL-5 or IL-4-induced eosinophilia. Omalizumab (Xolair) is a subcutaneously injected IgE antagonist (given every 2 to 4 weeks) that reduces asthma exacerbations by 25% in atopic patients. It has been shown to improve asthma-related quality of life, decrease mean daily rescue inhaler use, and reduce asthma symptoms in this subpopulation. Predictors of good response to omalizumab include F_{ENO} greater than 19.5 ppb, eosinophils greater than 260 per μL, or periostin greater than or equal to 50 ng/mL.[40] Mepolizumab (Nucala) is a subcutaneously injected IL-5 antagonist (given every 4 weeks) that reduces exacerbations by 50% and improves asthma-related quality of life in eosinophilic, exacerbation-prone patients.[41] It has also been shown to facilitate corticosteroid reduction in patients who are dependent on systemic steroids.[42] The likelihood of benefit increases with increasing antecedent exacerbation history and increasing serum eosinophil levels. Reslizumab (Cinqair) is an intravenous IL-5 antagonist (given every 4 weeks using weight-based dosing) that also reduces exacerbations by about 50% in eosinophilic patients.[43] Benralizumab (Fasenra) is a subcutaneous IL-5 receptor antagonist (given initially every 4 weeks and, after three doses, given every 8 weeks) that reduces asthma exacerbations and has a glucocorticoid-sparing effect in asthmatic patients with eosinophilia.[44] Dupilumab (Dupixent) is a subcutaneous IL-4 receptor antagonist (given every 2 weeks) that reduces exacerbations, has a steroid sparing effect, and improves lung function.[45]

Bronchial Thermoplasty

While bronchial thermoplasty is FDA-approved in severe asthma, international European Respiratory Society and American Thoracic Society guidelines suggest its use be restricted to international review board-approved clinical trials or registries.[46] Data on bronchial thermoplasty are limited mainly to trials without a sham procedure group, with only one trial including a sham arm.[26] There is moderate evidence that bronchial thermoplasty increases asthma exacerbations during the first year after treatment, but reduces exacerbations thereafter.[47] We generally support the use of bronchial thermoplasty in severe asthma that has failed the previously mentioned therapies (ie, in patients who do not meet criteria to receive biologic therapy or who have failed the biologics).

OTHER PULMONARY CAUSES OF COUGH

While asthma is frequently cited as the most common pulmonary cause of cough in persons with a normal or unremarkable chest radiograph, we acknowledge that most smokers generally do not seek medical attention for cough related to chronic bronchitis. Thus, even though chronic bronchitis accounts for about 5% of chronic cough in most series,[1] this is likely an underrepresentation of its true prevalence in the general population. Chronic bronchitis is mainly seen in current and former smokers, with a small subset seen in individuals who have airway inflammation from chronic inhalation of dusts or fumes. It causes a long-standing productive cough, usually of clear or white (mucoid) sputum.

Eosinophilic bronchitis is another common cause of chronic cough, accounting for 10% to 15% of cases presenting to a specialist clinic.[5] Eosinophilic bronchitis is defined by cough in patients with eosinophilic inflammation of the airway epithelium and no evidence of bronchoconstriction. Other pulmonary etiologies of cough include bronchiectasis (accounting for 4% of chronic cough in some series[1]), interstitial lung diseases, endobronchial tumors (carcinoid in particular), and lung cancers. In a person with long-standing, unexplained cough, a chest CT scan is indicated to evaluate for these pulmonary etiologies of cough that may not be identified on plain films of the chest.

THINKING OUTSIDE OF THE BOX

- We discourage the use of the term "reactive airways disease" in adults to describe a condition vaguely thought of as mild, transient asthma. We believe it represents imprecise thinking. Persons with and without asthma may experience a lingering cough following a respiratory tract infection. Persons without asthma have "postbronchitic cough" and, in the absence of severe bronchiolitis, normal lung function. Persons with asthma have variable airflow obstruction and all of the other pathologic features of asthma described above. Patients deserve to know whether they have the chronic medical condition, asthma, or normal airways with transient viral-induced cough; and providers have the means to make this distinction.

- The interaction between cough, asthma, and gastroesophageal reflux disease is multifaceted and complex. Cough and asthma may worsen esophageal reflux, and vice versa. Beyond dispute is recognition that the combination of laryngopharyngeal reflux together with oropharyngeal dysfunction and a predilection to aspiration can lead to prolonged cough, asthma attacks, aspiration pneumonia, and possible tracheal injury. On the other hand, the role esophageal reflux limited to the lower esophagus plays in aggravating asthma remains debated. A clinically useful study examined the effect of intense antiacid therapy with a proton-pump inhibitor on the course of poorly controlled asthma among persons free of gastrointestinal symptoms of reflux and found no benefit compared with placebo.[48] As a result, one focus in treating active asthma has been to inquire about and address the presence of *symptomatic* reflux, with the goal of alleviating gastrointestinal symptoms and possibly improving asthma control.

TAKE-HOME POINTS

- Persons with asthma may present with a persistent, troublesome cough without complaining of (or experiencing) other telltale symptoms of asthma, such as wheeze, shortness of breath, and chest tightness.
- The diagnosis of asthma may be suspected based on the characteristic triggers that provoke cough, such as exposure to a cat or dog, or on its timing, such as in the minutes following exercise, especially when performed in cold air.
- Cough due to asthma typically improves or resolves with treatment with bronchodilators and inhaled or oral corticosteroids. However, patients with cough due to other causes may also note improvement with these treatments; failure to improve with inhaled corticosteroids may reflect improper use of inhaled medications rather than an incorrect diagnosis.
- The diagnosis of asthma is best made by demonstration of variable airflow obstruction on pulmonary function testing, specifically spirometry. Persistent cough in a patient with airflow

obstruction that varies over time, that reverses acutely following administration of bronchodilator, or that can be elicited by provocative stimuli such as methacholine or exercise, can be presumed to be due, at least in part, to asthma.

- Effective treatments exist for asthma of all degrees of severity and should be applied in a stepwise fashion until good symptom control is achieved.

REFERENCES

1. Irwin RS, Curley FJ, French CL. Chronic cough: the spectrum and frequency of causes, key components of the diagnostic evaluation, and outline of specific therapy. *Am Rev Respir Dis*. 1990;141: 640–647.
2. Pratter MR, Bartter, T, Akers S, DuBois J. An algorithmic approach to chronic cough. *Ann Intern Med*. 1993;119:977–983.
3. McGarvey LP, Heaney LG, Lawson JT, et al. Evaluation and outcome of patients with chronic non-productive cough using a comprehensive diagnostic protocol. *Thorax*. 1998;53:738–743.
4. McFadden ER. Exertional dyspnea and cough as preludes to acute attacks of bronchial asthma. *New Engl J Med*. 1975;292:555–559.
5. Brightling CE, Ward R, Goh KL, Wardlaw AJ, Pavord ID. Eosinophilic bronchitis is an important cause of chronic cough. *Am J Respir Crit Care Med*. 1999;160: 406–410.
6. Fujimura M, Ogawa H, Nishizawa Y, Nishi K. Comparison of atopic cough with cough variant asthma: is atopic cough a precursor of asthma? *Thorax*. 2003;58: 14–18.
7. McFadden, ER Jr, Steven JB. History of asthma. In: Middleton E, Reed C, Ellis E, eds. *Allergy: Principles and Practice.* 2nd ed. St. Louis, MO: C V Mosby; 1983: 805–809.
8. Brightling CE, Bradding P, Symon FA, Holgate ST, Wardlaw, AJ, Pavord ID. Mast cell infiltration of airway smooth muscle in asthma. *N Engl J Med*. 2002; 346:1699–1705.
9. Siddiqui S, Mistry V, Doe C, et al. Airway hyperresponsiveness is dissociated from airway wall structural remodelling. *J Allergy Clin Immunol*. 2008;122:335–341.
10. Busse WW, Lemanske Jr RF. Asthma. *N Engl J Med*. 2001;344:350–362.
11. Dicpinigaitis PV. Chronic cough due to asthma. ACCP evidence-based clinical practice guidelines. *Chest*. 2006;129:75S–79S.
12. Komaki Y, Miura M, Takahashi M. Distribution of airway hyperresponsiveness in adult-onset cough-variant asthma: comparison with classic asthma. *Am J Respir Crit Care Med*. 2001;163:A419.
13. Moorman JE, Akinbami LJ, Bailey CM, et al. National Surveillance of Asthma: United States, 2001–2010. National Center for Health Statistics. *Vital Health Stat*. 2012;3(35).
14. Yunginger JW, Reed CE, O'Connell EJ, Melton LJ III, O'Fallon WM, Silverstein MD. A community-based study of the epidemiology of asthma. Incidence rates, 1964–1983. *Am Rev Respir Dis*. 1992;146:888–894.

15. Corrao WM, Braman SS, Irwin RS. Chronic cough as the sole presenting manifestation of bronchial asthma. *N Engl J Med*. 1979;300:633–637.
16. Koh YY, Jeong JH, Park Y, Kim, CK. Development of wheezing in patients with cough-variant asthma during an increase in airway responsiveness. *Eur Respir J*. 1999;14:302–308.
17. National Asthma Education and Prevention Program: Expert panel report 3: Guidelines for the diagnosis and management of asthma. National Heart, Lung, and Blood Institute. Bethesda, MD. (NIH publication no. 08-4051). http://www.nhlbi.nih.gov/guidelines/asthma/asthgdln.htm. Published 2007.
18. Korevaar DA, Westerhof GA, Wang J, et al. Diagnostic accuracy of minimally invasive markers for detection of airway eosinophilia in asthma: a systematic review and meta-analysis. *Lancet Respir Med*. 2015;3:290–300.
19. Smith AD, Cowan JO, Brassett KP, et al. Exhaled nitric oxide: a predictor of steroid response. *Am J Respir Crit Care Med*. 2005;172:453–459.
20. Aaron SD, Vandemheen KL, FitzGerald JM, et al. Reevaluation of diagnosis in adults with physician-diagnosed asthma. *J Amer Med Assoc*. 2017;317:269–279.
21. Fanta CH. Drug therapy. Asthma. *N Engl J Med*. 2009;360;1002–1014.
22. Nelson HS. β-Adrenergic bronchodilators. *N Engl J Med*. 1995;*333*:499–506.
23. Drazen JM, Israel E, Boushey HA, et al. Comparison of regularly scheduled with as-needed use of albuterol in mild asthma. *N Engl J Med*. 1996;335:841–847.
24. Busse WW, Dahl R, Jenkins C, Cruz AA. Long-acting muscarinic antagonists: a potential add-on therapy in the treatment of asthma? *Eur Respir Rev*. 2016;25: 54–64.
25. Gibson PG, Yang IA, Upham JW, et al. Effect of azithromycin on asthma exacerbations and quality of life in adults with persistent uncontrolled asthma (AMAZES): a randomised, double-blind, placebo-controlled trial. *Lancet*. 2017; 390:659–668.
26. Castro M, Rubin AS, Laviolette M, et al. Effectiveness and safety of bronchial thermoplasty in the treatment of severe asthma. *Am J Respir Crit Care Med*. 2010; 181:116–124.
27. Suissa S, Ernst P, Benayoun S, Baltzan M, Cai B. Low-dose inhaled corticosteroids and the prevention of death from asthma. *N Engl J Med*. 2000;343:332–336.
28. McKeever T, Mortimer K, Wilson A, et al. Quadrupling inhaled glucocorticoid dose to abort asthma exacerbations. *N Engl J Med*. 2018;378:902–910.
29. Chanez P, Bourdin A, Vachier I, Godard P, Bousquet J, Vignola AM. Effects of inhaled corticosteroids on pathology in asthma and chronic obstructive pulmonary disease. *Proc Am Thorac Soc*. 2004;1:184–190.
30. Lundgren R, Soderberg M, Horstedt P, Stenling R. Morphological studies of bronchial mucosal biopsies from asthmatics before and after ten years of treatment with inhaled steroids. *Eur Respir J*. 1988;1: 883–889.
31. Haahtela T, Jarvinen M, Kava T, et al. Comparison of a beta2-agonist, terbutaline, with an inhaled corticosteroid, budesonide, in newly detected asthma. *N Engl J Med*. 1991;325:388–392.
32. Sovijarvi AR, Haahtela T, Ekroos HJ, et al. Sustained reduction in bronchial hyperresponsiveness with inhaled fluticasone propionate within three days in mild asthma: time course after onset and cessation of treatment. *Thorax*. 2003; 58:500–504.
33. Lazarus SC, Boushey HA, Fahy JV, et al; Asthma Clinical Research Network for the National Heart, Lung, and Blood Institute. Long-acting beta2-agonist

monotherapy vs continued therapy with inhaled corticosteroids in patients with persistent asthma: a randomized controlled trial. *JAMA.* 2001;285:2583–2593.
34. Nelson HS, Weiss ST, Bleecker ER, Yancey SW, Dorinsky PM; SMART Study Group. The Salmeterol Multicenter Asthma Research Trial: a comparison of usual pharmacotherapy for asthma or usual pharmacotherapy plus salmeterol. *Chest.* 2006;129:15–26. [Erratum, *Chest*, 129:1393.]
35. Peters SP, Bleecker ER, Canonica GW, et al. Serious asthma events with budesonide plus formoterol vs budesonide alone. *N Engl J Med.* 2016;375:850–860.
36. Stempel DA, Raphiou IH, Kral KM, et al; AUSTRI Investigators. Serious asthma events with fluticasone plus salmeterol versus fluticasone alone. *N Engl J Med.* 2016;374:1822–1830.
37. Lazarus SC, Chinchilli VM, Rollings NJ, et al; National Heart Lung and Blood Institute's Asthma Clinical Research Network. Smoking affects response to inhaled corticosteroids or leukotriene receptor antagonists in asthma. *Am J Respir Crit Care Med.* 2007;175:783–790.
38. Peters-Golden M, Swern A, Bird SS, Hustad, CM, Grant E, Edelman JM. Influence of body mass index on the response to asthma controller agents. *Eur Respir J.* 2006;27:495–503.
39. Dahlen S, Malmström K, Nizankowska E, et al. Improvement of aspirin-intolerant asthma by montelukast, a leukotriene antagonist: a randomized, double-blind, placebo-controlled trial. *Am J Respir Crit Care Med.* 2002;165:9–14.
40. Hanania NA, Alpan O, Hamilos DL, et al. Omalizumab in severe allergic asthma inadequately controlled with standard therapy. A randomized trial. *Ann Intern Med.* 2011;154:573–582.
41. Pavord ID, Korn S, Howarth P, et al. Mepolizumab for severe eosinophilic asthma (DREAM): a multicenter, double-blind, placebo-controlled trial. *Lancet,* 2012;380(9842):651–659.
42. Bel EH, Wenzel SE, Thompson PJ, et al; SIRIUS Investigators. Oral glucocorticoid-sparing effect of mepolizumab in eosinophilic asthma. *N Engl J Med.* 2014;371:1189–1197.
43. Castro M, Mathur S, Hargreave F, et al; Res-5-0010 Study Group. Reslizumab for poorly controlled, eosinophilic asthma: a randomized, placebo-controlled study. *Am J Respir Crit Care Med.* 2011;184:1125–1132.
44. Bleecker ER, FitzGerald JM, Chanez P, et al; SIROCCO study investigators. Efficacy and safety of benralizumab for patients with severe asthma uncontrolled with high-dosage inhaled corticosteroids and long-acting β2-agonists (SIROCCO): a randomised, multicentre, placebo-controlled phase 3 trial. *Lancet.* 2016;388:2115–2127.
45. Castro M, Corren J, Pavord ID, et al. (2018). Dupilumab efficacy and safety in moderate-to-severe uncontrolled asthma. *N Engl J Med.* 2016;378;2486
46. Chung KF, Wenzel SE, Brozek JL. International ERS/ATS guidelines on definition, evaluation and treatment of severe asthma. *Eur Respir J.* 2014;43(2):343–373
47. Torrego A, Sola I, Munoz AM, et al. Bronchial thermoplasty for moderate or severe persistent asthma in adults. *Cochrane Database Syst Rev,* 2014;(3): CD009910. Retrieved from https://www.ncbi.nlm.nih.gov/pubmed/24585221
48. Mastronarde JG, Anthonisen NR, Castro M, et al. Efficacy of esomeprazole for treatment of poorly controlled asthma. *N Engl J Med.* 2009;360:1487–1499.

3

SINONASAL DISEASE AND ALLERGY AS AN ETIOLOGY OF CHRONIC COUGH

Alice Z. Maxfield and Benjamin S. Bleier

INTRODUCTION

Cough may be of multifactorial etiology, and can manifest as a bothersome symptom or a predominant sign of serious airway diseases. The diagnosis of cough is often a diagnosis of exclusion. Published guidelines on cough management have been criticized for their basis on expert opinion rather than high-quality evidence. Nevertheless, there is a plethora of literature on the diagnosis and management of cough, which is helpful in confronting this common and challenging problem.

The most common causes of cough include gastroesophageal reflux disease (GERD), asthma syndromes, and disorders of the upper airway; therefore, both pulmonary and extrapulmonary causes for chronic cough must be considered.[1] There is an abundance of literature supporting the connection between the upper and lower airway and how disorders of the upper airway, such as sinonasal disease, can be a contributing source of chronic cough. This chapter will focus on the relationship between the upper and lower airway and discuss upper airway diseases that include cough as a major symptom.

UNIFIED AIRWAY

Patients frequently present to multiple specialties, including their primary care physician, otolaryngologist, and pulmonologist, for workup of respiratory tract complaints. Knowledge and familiarity of the coexistence of upper and lower airway inflammatory conditions are essential in the diagnosis and management of these diseases. Both epidemiologic and pathophysiologic studies have established the connection between the upper and lower airway, supporting the concept of a unified system. The "unified airway model" describes the need for evaluation of the entire respiratory tract from the nose and paranasal sinuses to the trachea and distal bronchioles as one integrated entity. Symptoms arise from the upper airway secondary to allergic and nonallergic rhinitis and from the lower airway as related to asthma. However, one inflammatory condition can initiate a response from another part of the respiratory system, instigating a new response or exacerbating one that is already present. Local and systemic stimuli generate an inflammatory process throughout the upper and lower airway, exacerbating symptoms or creating resistance to treatment if not all systems are addressed. The overall severity of the disease and treatment of each may affect the overall improvement in symptoms and control of the disease process. As such, a thoughtful approach that encompasses and considers the entire airway, including potential extra-airway insult from the alimentary tract, should be taken when evaluating and treating the patient with cough.[2]

Relationship Between the Upper and Lower Airway: Epidemiologic Evidence

Epidemiologic studies have established the relationship between upper airway diseases, specifically rhinitis and rhinosinusitis, and lower airway illnesses, such as asthma, supporting the unified airway model. Rhinitis and rhinosinusitis confer a significant health burden on the overall population. The prevalence of allergic rhinitis ranges from 15% to 40% and is the fifth most common chronic disease in the United States.[3–5] Rhinosinusitis affects 12% of adults in the US population and is the number one diagnosis leading to an antibiotic prescription.[6] Research has proven that rhinitis is a primary risk factor in the development of asthma and that there is an increase in bronchial hyperresponsiveness in rhinitis patients. Therefore, otolaryngologists and specialists need to be aware of this association between the upper and lower airway to properly diagnose and manage these illnesses and to optimize treatment outcomes.

Rhinitis and asthma frequently coexist, and upper airway inflammation often precedes lower airway disease. Studies have shown that nasal symptoms occur in up to 78% of patients with asthma. Up to 38% of patients with allergic rhinitis and nonallergic rhinitis also have asthma.[7–11] Compared to patients with no history of either disease, there was a two- to fourfold higher incidence of new diagnosis of allergic rhinitis or asthma in patients who previously had one of these diseases.[11–12] There is also a temporal relationship between the development of rhinitis and asthma. It has been shown that 64% of patients had rhinitis before the onset of asthma, and 21% had both upper and lower airway disease at the same time.[11,13] In another study, 49% of patients had nasal symptoms first and 25% had both diseases within 1 year of each other.[9,11] These findings demonstrate that nasal symptoms of allergic rhinitis precede the development of lower airway symptoms, and patients have an increased risk of developing asthma over time.[2] Yawn et al found that the association of asthma and allergic rhinitis varied with the age of first diagnosis of asthma, which may demonstrate a relationship between allergic rhinitis and asthma triggers, such as exposure to allergens.[14] Therefore, it is unclear if what causes nasal symptoms leads to the first manifestation of the airway disease process or if the nasal symptoms themselves lead to the development of lower airway disease. Regardless, the association between the two demonstrates the need to evaluate the airway as a unified entity.

Additionally, the presence of allergic rhinitis is a risk factor in the severity of asthma and, conversely, the severity of nasal symptoms has been found to correlate to the severity of asthma.[2,15] Total medical care and respiratory care cost was significantly higher when patients had both asthma and allergic rhinitis as compared to asthma alone.[14] Therefore, proper diagnosis and treatment of rhinitis may prevent the development of asthma and improve asthma control.

Chronic rhinosinusitis (CRS) is a significant burden on direct and indirect health care costs with substantial impact on quality of life. It is currently classified by clinical phenotype, although there is a wide spectrum of presentations with overlap in symptoms. CRS is most commonly grouped into CRS with nasal polyps (CRSwNP) and CRS without nasal polyps (CRSsNP), but can also be divided based on the inflammatory state—eosinophilic versus neutrophilic. Eosinophilic rhinosinusitis is the category of upper airway disease most associated with asthma. It presents with thick mucus production, nasal congestion, loss of smell, and acute bacterial exacerbations. The pathophysiology is based on the secretion of cytokines, specifically interleukin-5 (IL-5), which promotes the accumulation of eosinophils in the sinonasal mucosa, causing inflammation and symptoms. Patients with CRS have a 20% prevalence of asthma as compared to 5% to 8% in the general population.[16] In those patients with CRSwNP, the prevalence of asthma increases to 50%.[17] Treatment of CRS with medical therapy and surgical intervention has been shown to improve asthma control and decrease asthma medication usage. Additionally, surgical treatment of nasal polyps has been shown to have long-term improvement in lower airway disease.[17] Based on these epidemiologic studies, the coexistence of asthma and CRS, particularly the eosinophilic subtype, has been recognized and further evaluated to prove the connection from histopathologic findings.

NONALLERGIC RHINITIS AND ASTHMA

Most studies have focused on the relationship between allergic rhinitis and asthma; however, nonallergic rhinitis is also strongly associated with asthma. Nonallergic rhinitis can be divided into nonallergic rhinitis without eosinophilia (aka vasomotor rhinitis) or nonallergic rhinitis with eosinophilia (NARES). In a study using a questionnaire, measurement of total and specific immunoglobulin IgE, allergy skin-prick tests, and bronchoprovocation challenges with methacholine, asthma was strongly associated with both allergic and nonallergic rhinitis and remained highly significant when the analysis was limited to nonatopic subjects with relatively low IgE levels.[18] All rhinitis was found to be a significant risk factor for asthma, and increased the risk of developing asthma by threefold.[19]

Clinical Relationship Between Rhinitis and Asthma

Airway inflammation in asthma, which leads to the symptomology, is triggered by the activation of eosinophils, mast cells, and T lymphocytes. It has been demonstrated that clinical severity, airway hyperresponsiveness, and lung function are related mainly to eosinophilic inflammation.[20] Additionally, the infiltration with T-helper lymphocytes expressing Th2-type cytokines in nasal and bronchial mucosa are well documented in both allergic asthma and rhinitis.[21,22] These cytokine mediators are responsible for the vascular engorgement and mucosal edema that cause the symptoms of rhinitis, including nasal obstruction, sneezing, and rhinorrhea. This inflammatory cascade also correlates with the severity of asthma symptoms and degree of bronchial hyperresponsiveness.[21] Based on this, nasal allergies may induce lower airway responsiveness, despite the lack of a formal diagnosis of asthma, leading to the concept of increased asthma susceptibility in those with rhinitis and suggesting that rhinitis and asthma are one disease process that manifests in different parts of the airway system.

In the presence of severe rhinitis, patients with asthma are associated with a worse prognosis and require more asthma treatment.[23,24] Additionally, those patients with allergic rhinitis without a diagnosis of asthma also show bronchospasm and hyperresponsiveness, especially with nasal allergy challenge.[25] In a survey from the European Community Respiratory Health Survey, self-reported "nasal allergies" were an independent predictor of bronchial hyperreactivity.[26] The difference between perennial allergies and seasonal allergies also alters the degree of hyperresponsiveness. Prieto et al found a lower methacholine threshold value and higher level of plateau on bronchial provocation testing in those with perennial allergies as compared to those with seasonal allergies.[4] Nonasthmatics usually reach a maximal response plateau at a mild degree of airway narrowing as compared to patients with asthma, who do not reach a plateau response, leading to increased airway narrowing. In combination with the epidemiologic relationship between rhinitis and asthma, this demonstrates a strong correlation between the two diseases.

As further evidence strengthening the unified airway model, studies have shown therapeutic effects of rhinitis treatment on asthma. Intranasal corticosteroids prevent increases in nonspecific bronchial reactivity and asthma symptoms associated with seasonal pollen exposure.[11] Specifically, in a 4-week trial of intranasal budesonide in patients with perennial nasal allergy and asthma, not only was chronic nasal obstruction improved, but daily asthma symptoms and exercise-induced bronchospasm were also reduced.[11] Studies have also found more effective improvement in bronchial responsiveness with intranasal delivery of corticosteroid as compared to oral inhalation.[27] This demonstrates that intranasal delivery of corticosteroids is effective in managing lower airway symptoms in patients with allergic rhinitis.

Clinical Relationship Between Chronic Rhinosinusitis and Asthma

Eosinophilic-mediated or T-helper (Th) 2 type inflammation leading to CRSwNP is the subtype most commonly associated with asthma, particularly late-onset asthma.[28] Based on histopathologic findings, eosinophil infiltration and similar airway remodeling are found throughout the upper and lower airway. Basement membrane thickening, goblet cell hyperplasia, subepithelial edema, mucus hypersecretion, and epithelial damage are among the common findings in both the upper and lower airways in CRS and asthma.[28–32] Th2 lymphocytes trigger the release of cytokines IL-4, IL-5, and IL-13, which are inflammatory mediators that drive the cascade leading to both upper airway symptoms and lower-airway inflammation.

Clinical studies have used symptoms and computed tomography (CT) imaging to identify the correlation between CRS and asthma. There is a highly significant correlation between extent of sinus involvement based on CT imaging and the severity of asthma.[33] Eosinophil count in peripheral blood was also directly correlated with symptom scores and sinus CT imaging scores in those with mild to moderate asthma. Therefore, this leads to the conclusion that rhinosinusitis and asthma are the manifestations of eosinophilic inflammatory process in the upper and lower airways. Brinke et al also found CT imaging abnormalities in those with severe asthma, even in the absence of nasal symptoms. These findings were more frequently associated with adult-onset asthma, indicating the eosinophil mediated inflammatory process is the driver of both upper and lower airway diseases.[28,34] The medical and surgical treatment of CRS is associated with improvement in asthma, which further supports the hypothesis that inflammation of the upper airway has direct effects on the lower airway through inflammatory mediators and cytokines.

Clinical Relationship Between Chronic Rhinosinusitis and Laryngopharyngeal Reflux

GERD or laryngopharyngeal reflux (LPR) has been linked to multiple disease processes in the upper airway and middle ear.[35–40] In the pediatric population, LPR has been implicated as a reason for failure of CRS to respond to appropriate medical therapy.[35–37] In adults, CRS has been found to occur in greater frequency in patients with LPR than in those without, and those with medically refractory CRS have been found to be associated with higher likelihood of LPR.[38,41–43] Additionally, patients with persistent CRS after endoscopic sinus surgery were found to have more reflux at the distal and proximal aerodigestive tract, specifically the nasopharynx, representing a causative factor of refractory CRS that needs to be addressed.[44] GERD has also been found to be a significant predictor of poor symptomatic outcome after endoscopic sinus surgery for CRS.[45] Recent systematic review and meta-analysis also supported a significant association between GERD and CRS, and CRS patients were found to have a greater prevalence of intranasal *Helicobacter pylori* and acid reflux than those without CRS.[40] Although the exact pathophysiology of how LPR contributes to CRS is unknown, there is sufficient evidence supporting the effects of reflux on CRS, and consideration for treatment of both is recommended.

Pathophysiology of Upper and Lower Airway Interrelationship

The unified airway model is well supported; however, the pathophysiology connecting the upper and lower airway is poorly understood. There are several theories that explain the relationship between the upper and lower airway.[11] The first is the nasal–bronchial reflex, which describes trigeminal afferent nerves originating in the nose (afferent limb) causing efferent bronchoconstriction of the lower airway. Nasal stimulus with allergens has been shown to cause lower airway resistance, such as with silica,[4] nasal petrolatum packing,[47] and cold air.[48] Between 11% and 32% of patients with rhinitis have positive bronchoconstrictor responses to histamine, methacholine, or carbachol in the range of responses consistent with patients with asthma.[11,49–51] It has also been shown that exposure of cold air to the nasal mucosa induces a positive bronchoconstrictor response in normal individuals.[52] The effect is attributed to the cholinergic reflex because the systemic administration of atropine[46] and resection of the trigeminal nerve[53] have been shown to prevent this bronchospasm (efferent limb).

The second theory describes the shift from nasal to mouth breathing with nasal obstruction, leading to bronchospasm. Improvement in lower airway symptoms may be the result of better humidification and warming of the air with nasal breathing, preventing lower airway constriction.

The third theory is the aspiration of sinonasal drainage. Several animal studies have identified upper respiratory tract substances in the tracheobronchial tree, and the blockage of this has prevented nonspecific bronchial responsiveness.[54–56] Nelson et al performed a prospective study evaluating pulmonary aspirates and identified aspiration of sinonasal secretions into the lungs of both patients with cystic fibrosis and healthy adults in the recumbent position.[57]

The theory of systemic amplification has also been used to explain the linkage between CRS and asthma. This describes that one airway compartment can impact disease in another through inflammatory mediators and the recruitment of these inflammatory progenitors from the peripheral blood to the airway.[15] Thus, control of one airway compartment leads to the improvement of symptoms in another airway compartment, such as with control of CRS and associated improvement in asthma.

The unified airway model considers multiple facets of airway disease to elucidate the connection between upper airway disease, such as rhinitis and rhinosinusitis, and asthma. The evidence behind this model supports the need to consider the upper and lower airway together, both for diagnosis and for treatment to optimize outcome. The prevalence of rhinitis and rhinosinusitis in asthmatic patients demonstrate that these are different manifestations of respiratory disease within one system.[15] The exact pathogenesis of how upper airway disease leads to lower airway disease is unknown; however, this review of the literature supporting the unified airway model highlights the importance of being familiar with these common conditions for diagnosis and management of the symptom chronic cough.

WHEN IT ISN'T SINONASAL DISEASE

When smoking and angiotensin converting enzyme (ACE) inhibitor use are ruled out as a cause for chronic cough, three diagnoses account for more than 90% of all chronic cough symptoms: cough-variant asthma (CVA), GERD or LPR, or postnasal drip (PND).[58,59] In 2006, the American College of Chest Physicians updated its evidence-based guidelines on cough and replaced the diagnosis of postnasal drip syndrome (PNDS) with upper airway cough syndrome (UACS). Although a significant amount of idiopathic chronic cough is attributed to postnasal drip, the diagnosis of PND lacks objective diagnostic measures and is based on highly variable symptoms as described by patients. UACS can be caused by various types of rhinitis, as described below. The mechanism of how PND induces cough is controversial and largely unproven. The pharyngobronchial reflex hypothesizes that the mechanical drainage of secretions from the sinonasal tract into the hypopharynx causes pharyngeal constriction, and ultimately bronchoconstriction and cough symptoms.[19] PND is described as the drainage of secretions from the nose and paranasal sinuses into the pharynx that is eventually swallowed.[59] This is reported by patients as a sensation of "something dripping down the back of the throat," sore throat in the morning, and frequent spitting of mucus. The direct visualization of mucus or secretions in the posterior pharynx is unreliable and there may not be evidence of nasal secretions, termed "silent PND."[58] Other signs on physical examination include cobblestoning of the posterior pharyngeal mucosa or swollen mucous glands. Pratter et al demonstrated that 20% of the chronic cough patients diagnosed with PND were asymptomatic from the drainage, such as throat clearing and sensation of PND, and 59% of these patients had negative physical exam findings, such as nasal secretions and cobblestoning of the posterior pharynx.[60] Therefore, this leads to the controversy of the pathogenesis of chronic cough from UACS.

One explanation of cough from UACS is the direct irritation by nasal secretions in the larynx and pharynx. However, O'Hara and Jones demonstrated that only 8% of patients with purulent nasal drainage had cough with no other pathology, thereby putting the hypothesis of direct irritation by secretions in question.[61] More recent work has explored the phenomenon of increased sensitivity of cough reflex secondary to an insult, causing hyperresponsiveness of cough receptors. Studies looking at the effects of capsaicin has suggested that chronic cough may be secondary to decreased threshold of the cough reflex in those with UACS as compared to those with rhinitis/sinusitis without cough and healthy patients.[62] Additionally, cough reflex sensitivity has been shown to have transient hyperresponsiveness induced by upper respiratory infection, leading to the concept of hypersensitivity as an explanation for chronic cough.[63] Allergens and irritants stimulate the afferent limb of the cough reflex peripherally, leading to central reactivity that manifests as cough.[59] In the setting of chronic cough without evidence of PND or allergic symptoms with a normal intranasal exam, GERD and LPR are presumed the etiology of chronic cough until proven otherwise.

Allergic rhinitis (AR) affects between 10% and 30% of the United States adult population, and 40% of children, making it the fifth most common chronic disease.[64] It is an inflammatory, IgE-mediated process characterized by nasal congestion, rhinorrhea, sneezing, and/or nasal itching with findings of sinonasal mucosal inflammation with exposure to specific allergens.[5] AR can be seasonal or perennial, and diagnosed with skin testing. The allergic response can be divided into early- and late-phase symptoms, with early-phase symptoms including sneezing, pruritus, and rhinorrhea, while congestion is predominantly a late-phase reaction. If an allergic reaction to specific antigens is identified on skin testing, a positive treatment response may lead to the diagnosis of AR as the cause for UACS.

Nonallergic rhinitis (NAR) is classified by the presence of similar chronic nasal symptoms in the absence of IgE-mediated response and with negative skin testing. NAR can be classified into inflammatory and noninflammatory etiologies. Inflammatory NAR includes postinfectious rhinitis, NARES, and nonallergic rhinitis with nasal polyps. Noninflammatory nonallergic rhinitis includes vasomotor rhinitis, rhinitis medicamentosa, rhinitis of pregnancy, rhinitis due to physical or chemical irritants, and rhinitis due to anatomic abnormalities of the sinonasal tract, such as deviated nasal septum, inferior turbinate hypertrophy, and maxillary sinus recirculation. NAR can lead to UACS and ultimately a chronic cough through mechanisms similar to that of AR.

NARES is also a diagnosis of exclusion with similar but more intense symptoms, including perennial sneezing, pruritus of nasal and ocular mucosa, and excessive lacrimation. The diagnosis is based on negative skin testing, absence of serum IgE antibodies to allergens, and elevated eosinophils in nasal secretions.[59]

Vasomotor rhinitis accounts for most of NAR and is described as the overactive nose involving an autonomic nervous system dysfunction, characterized by predominance of the parasympathetic system, leading to nasal secretions, vasodilation, and edema of the sinonasal mucosa.[59,64,65] Symptoms of rhinorrhea (e.g., nasal congestion and postnasal drip) leading to UACS and cough can be triggered by various stimuli, such as change in temperature, strong odors, respiratory irritants, emotional stress, spicy foods, and alcoholic beverages.[65]

Postinfectious UACS, also known as postviral vagal neuropathy (PVVN), is diagnosed based on the symptoms of chronic cough preceded by a recent history of viral or bacterial upper respiratory tract infection when the cough is present 8 weeks or more after resolution of other symptoms. Hypersensitivity of the cough reflex is a well-known phenomenon; however, in a subset of patients, this hypersensitivity persists and becomes a chronic cough. Studies have shown that cough reflex sensitivity is transiently enhanced during acute viral URI compared with the postrecovery state.[66] Based on similar findings, the newly proposed cough hypersensitivity syndrome has been suggested as a concept explaining chronic cough. It is based on the mechanism of dysregulated sensory neural functions triggered by low-level stimuli.[67,68] Viral infections, such as herpes simplex virus and influenza virus, and other irritants can cause local inflammation and injury of vagal nerves, leading to central pathway dysfunction and cough hypersensitivity.[68] See Chapter 6 for more information on neurogenic cough.

Rhinitis medicamentosa is described as severe rebound swelling of the nasal mucosa secondary to chronic use of nasal decongestants. Patients become dependent on the use of the topical decongestants to relieve nasal congestion and, over time, require more frequent application in larger doses. Treatment requires discontinuing the use of the nasal decongestant, which may be difficult for patients because of the rebound nasal blockage ensuing from the chronic use. The use of nasal steroid spray has been used to help patients wean off of the topical decongestant.

Rhinitis of pregnancy, or hormonal rhinitis, is nasal congestion from mucosal swelling resulting from increased circulating blood volume and vasodilation caused by hormones, leading to vascular pooling and edema, secondary to leakage of plasma from the vascular bed into the stroma.[69] There are limited clinical trials in the use of intranasal corticosteroid spray in pregnancy. However, based on the current literature, fluticasone, mometasone, and budesonide are safe when used at the recommended dosage.[70]

Rhinitis due to chemical or environmental irritants and occupational rhinitis is described as noninflammatory rhinitis with symptoms of nasal congestion, rhinorrhea, sneezing, and itching following exposure to irritants in the environment. Diagnosis depends on a thorough history with a temporal relationship between exposure and onset of symptoms. Treatment includes avoidance and reduction in exposure of the irritant.

Anatomic abnormalities including deviated nasal septum, concha bullosa, and Haller cells have been implicated in the development of chronic rhinosinusitis[71–74] (Figure 3–1).

Alkire and Bhattacharyya identified that only Haller cells were related to the occurrence of recurrent acute rhinosinusitis.[75] Calhoun et al compared CT findings between those with sinus disease and healthy patients and found that septal deviation was associated with osteomeatal complex disease, anterior ethmoid, and posterior ethmoid disease.[76] Furthermore, the

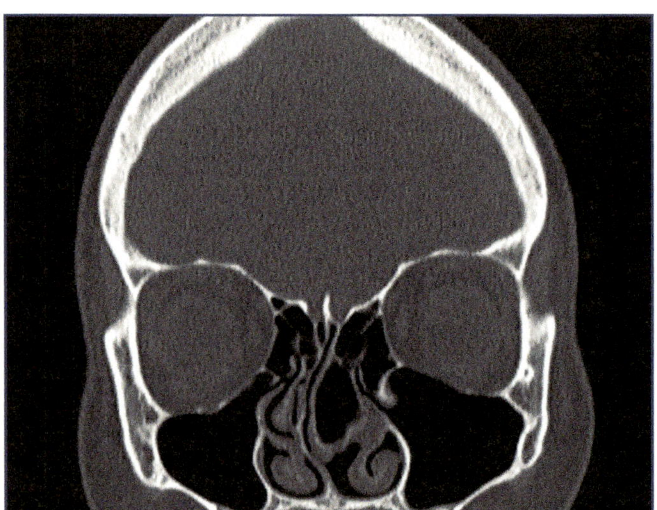

Figure 3–1. Coronal CT image showing a large left concha bullosa with severely deviated nasal septum to the right, and nasal polyp at the lateral aspect, which can contribute to postnasal drainage.

presence of concha bullosa was associated with anterior ethmoid disease. Dental pathology has also been associated with postnasal drainage and cough. One study showed a significant correlation between number of missing posterior teeth and postnasal drip and nasal congestion.[7] Additionally, obstruction of the maxillary sinus meatus and thickening of the maxillary sinus mucosa was associated with the complaint of cough.[77] Nasopharyngitis, adenoiditis, adenoid hypertrophy, Thornwaldt's cyst, and iatrogenic disease, such as maxillary sinus accessories causing mucous recirculation, can also contribute to postnasal drainage[78–81] (Figures 3–2 and 3–3).

Multiple chemical sensitivity (MCS), first identified in 1989, is defined as a multisystem disorder caused by exposure to environmental contaminants at concentrations below levels considered toxic for the general population, leading to symptoms involving multiple organ systems.[82,83] The presentation of MCS may be highly variable among individuals, ranging from mild occasional symptoms to severe debilitating symptoms. Symptoms can involve various sensory pathways, such as olfactory, trigeminal, gustatory, auditory, and visual, in response to exposure.[82] Although difficult to diagnose because of the variability of the condition and significant diversity of symptoms, it is important to be aware of the condition and how it may manifest as complaints of cough or upper respiratory symptoms.

Each of these conditions can be a source leading to chronic cough along with other symptoms. Diagnosis of each of these includes a thorough history from the patient and clinical examination to determine the cause of rhinitis leading to PND or UACS.

DIAGNOSIS

Based on review of the literature over the last 20 to 30 years, there are three main causes of cough. Common teaching of causes of cough, such as cigarette smoking and angiotensin-converting enzyme (ACE) inhibitor use, actually makes up but a small subset of patients.[58] In the majority of patients, the presence of one or any combination of these conditions is the likely cause of the chronic cough: UACS, asthma, and laryngopharyngeal reflux disease (LPRD) or GERD.[58] The asthma category includes cough-variant asthma, atopic cough, and eosinophilic bronchitis.[84] The American College of Chest Physicians (ACCP) consensus panel introduced UACS in 2006, which includes what was previously termed PNDS. Understanding the common causes for cough and consideration of both pulmonary and extrapulmonary causes is important for a thorough workup and diagnosis.

Guidelines for common conditions in otolaryngology and pulmonology, such as management of allergic rhinitis, chronic rhinosinusitis, asthma, and chronic obstructive pulmonary disease (COPD), have been shown to improve patient care and provide economic benefit.[1,85] The highly anticipated ACCP cough guidelines came out in 2006. However, they were met with criticism because of recommendations based more on opinion

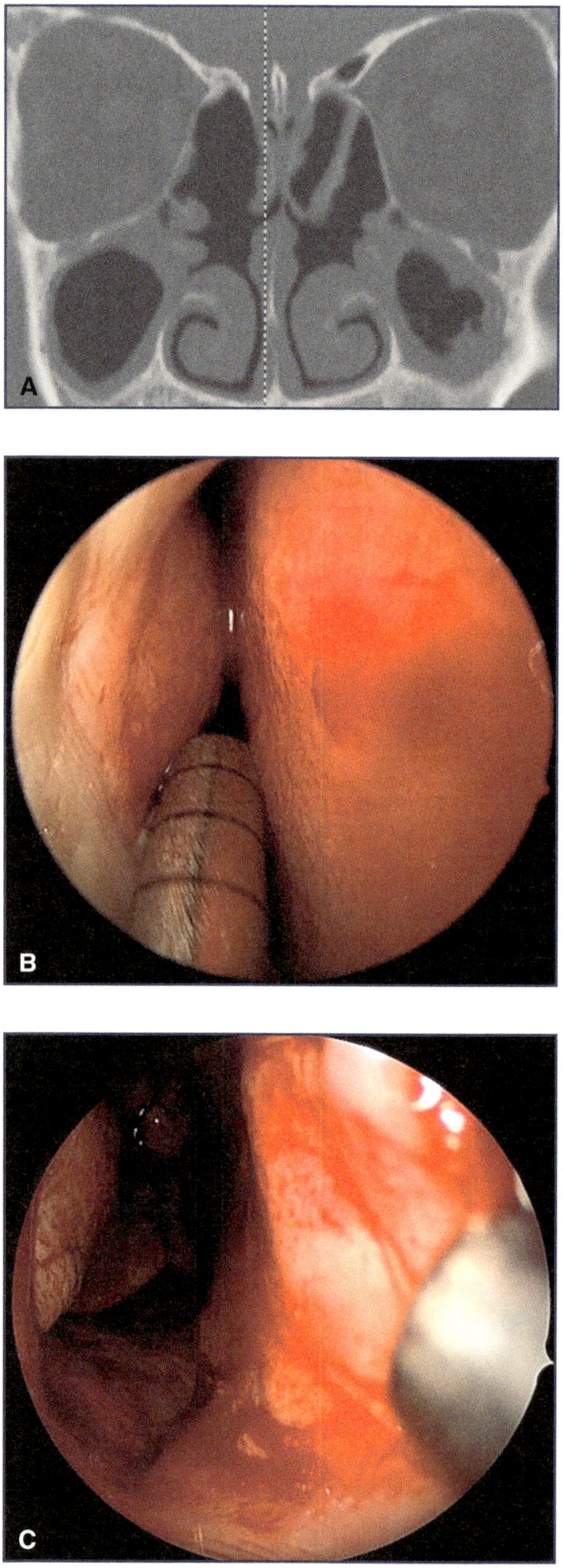

Figure 3–2. A. Inferior turbinate hypertrophy with chronic rhinosinusitis, specifically the maxillary sinus (shown here), can be a source of postnasal drainage leading to cough. **B.** Endoscopic preoperative photo of the right nasal passageway showing inferior turbinate hypertrophy. **C.** Endoscopic postoperative view of inferior turbinate submucosal reduction and lateralization to improve the right nasal airway, reduce nasal congestion, and decrease postnasal drainage.

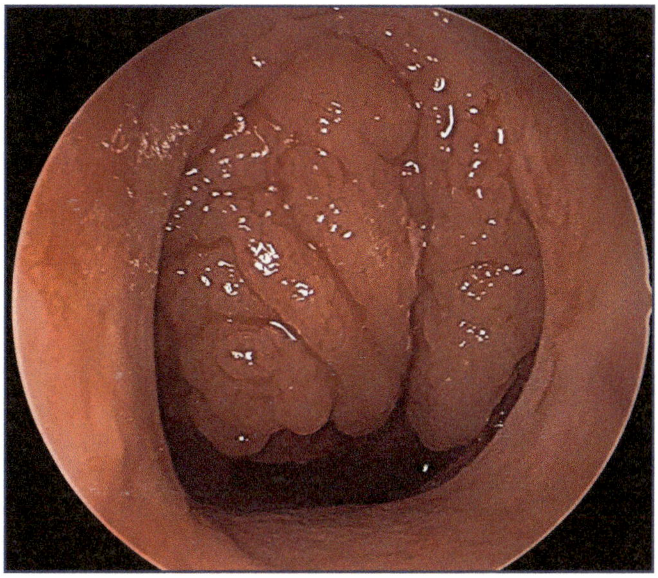

Figure 3–3. This is an endoscopic view of the left posterior nasal cavity with significant adenoid hypertrophy obstructing the nasopharynx, which can be a cause of postnasal drainage.

rather than evidence, with one-third of the recommendations based on "low" evidence and another one-quarter based on expert opinion only.[86–88] Despite this, the guidelines highlight the common causes for cough, treatment steps, and common reasons for treatment failures that help guide the clinician through this difficult and very common problem.

A detailed medical history with focus on sinonasal complaints is the initial step in identification of the underlying cause of chronic cough as it relates to the upper respiratory tract. Preceding events, such as recent upper respiratory and sinus infections, postnasal drip symptoms, aggravating factors, recent medications, and smoking history, are helpful in narrowing down possible etiologies and may help in determining treatment strategy. It is important to consider asymptomatic or "silent" UACS as a causative factor if questioning does not lead to a specific diagnosis.[60] UACS can be asymptomatic or present with complaints of sensation of something draining into the throat, throat clearing, tickle in throat, nasal congestion, or nasal discharge. A preceding event, such as upper respiratory illness, may be associated with the start of symptoms. Additionally, patients may not be aware of the relationship between symptoms or environmental factors that may precipitate the symptom of cough. Therefore, comprehensive questioning targeted to the upper respiratory tract is essential, and as stated earlier, reflux may be a contributing factor.

Clinical examination of the upper respiratory tract may be notable for positive findings in identifying contributing causes. A thorough examination of the nose with nasal endoscopy looking for obstruction, drainage, edema, and anatomical variants that may trigger postnasal drip can be helpful. The nasopharynx should be carefully evaluated for adenoid hypertrophy, cysts, and thick postnasal discharge. The oropharynx should be examined for signs of postnasal drip, such as posterior pharyngeal wall cobblestoning, drainage in the oropharynx, and characteristics of the sputum. The quality and quantity of sputum production should also be analyzed for possible bacterial growth, indicating sinusitis. It should be noted that many of these signs can be transient and not appreciated at the exact time of exam; however, presence of this can lead to decision making on treatment strategy. Auscultation of the upper airway for wheeze, stridor, and stertor can also direct further diagnostic testing. Based on previous studies, one-quarter of patients will have two causes for chronic cough, and PNDS is the cause nearly half the time.[89]

Following the initial assessment, imaging may also be a useful adjunct to corroborate positive or negative findings on exam and endoscopy. Sinus roentgenograms have mostly fallen out of favor; however, CT imaging of the sinuses should be considered to rule out chronic rhinosinusitis and other sinonasal pathologies, including anatomical variants that could contribute to symptoms. If history and clinical examination corroborate negative findings within the upper airway, then consideration must be given to GERD and LPR as the cause for the chronic cough.

TREATMENT

Based on the most common causes of chronic cough, several algorithms have been proposed in the treatment strategy. UACS, secondary to chronic, postviral, allergic, or vasomotor rhinitis, has been determined to be the most common cause of chronic cough.[58,60,89,90] Therefore, empiric treatment for UACS has been proposed prior to further testing and workup.[59] If there is a known trigger for UACS, the treatment can be focused on managing the specific condition. However, when the specific etiology of postnasal drip causing UACS is not clear, evidence-based empiric therapy should be trialed, because improvement in cough in response to treatment is the essential element in diagnosing UACS as a cause of cough.[59] Pratter et al showed that 59% of patients responded to first-generation antihistamine-decongestant therapy alone and 33% responded to antihistamine-decongestant therapy plus nasal corticosteroids.[60] Treatment of postnasal drip can resolve the cough even if underlying asthma is present.[60] Therefore, first-line treatment for UACS of unknown origin is empirical trial of first-generation antihistamine/decongestant,[59] such as diphenhydramine, chlorpheniramine, brompheniramine, and hydroxyzine, and/or intranasal corticosteroids.[91,92] Both first- and second-generation antihistamines are competitive antagonists to histamine at the H1-receptor site. However, most studies on cough suppression are based on the evaluation of the first-generation antihistamines because of their anticholinergic activity. Second-generation antihistamines, such as loratidine, terfenadine, and fexofenadine, have not been found to affect the cough reflex in the healthy patient or during an URI.[93–100]

Nasal steroid spray is the most effective therapy in controlling the nasal symptoms of allergic rhinitis by reducing secretory activity and mucosal inflammation, thereby reducing postnasal drip and cough.[91,92,101] Mometasone nasal spray once a day was found to be effective in relieving daytime cough severity, in addition to the nasal symptoms of seasonal allergic rhinitis.[92] If no response to empiric antihistamine/decongestant therapy with first-generation antihistamines and/or nasal steroids, sinus imaging should be considered to evaluate for further occult sinus pathology.[86]

In the absence of clinical disease, an empiric trial of ipratropium bromide nasal spray can also be trialed. A small prospective trial evaluated the treatment with fluticasone, ipratropium, and azelastine nasal spray on patients with chronic cough and postnasal drainage sensation and found improvement in nasal symptoms, endoscopic nasal scores, and cough.[102] Patients with postviral cough treated with placebo or a combination of nebulized salbutamol and ipratropium bromide were found to have an improvement in daytime and nighttime cough severity.[103] Most studies over the last 20 years have used inhaled anticholinergics, such as tiotropium, ipratropium, and oxitropium in patients with postviral cough syndrome or acute URI, which gave contradictory results.[104–106] However, the anticholinergic activity has been shown to inhibit mucous gland secretion, airway vessel dilation, and local mediator release, all of which contribute to upper airway symptoms during URI and allergic rhinitis. Therefore, an empiric trial of ipratropium bromide nasal spray may reduce cough symptoms associated with UACS. However, randomized controlled studies are needed to further elucidate this.[107]

Topical treatments allow directed local treatment while avoiding systemic side effects. Saline irrigations have been shown to significantly improve clinical symptoms and quality of life.[108–110] Topical saline solutions are promoted in the management of allergic rhinitis, chronic rhinosinusitis, and in postoperative care after endoscopic sinus surgery. Saline irrigations allow high-volume lavage of the sinonasal cavity thereby removing debris, allergens, and inflammatory markers that may escalate the inflammatory response. These rinses also serve to mechanically eliminate excess mucus that may lead to postnasal drainage and cough.

Xylitol is an organic sugar alcohol used in intranasal irrigations. It reduces salt concentration of the airway which enhances innate antimicrobial activity,[111] has antibiofilm properties,[112] and increases the concentration of microbiocidal nitric oxide.[113] Weissman et al found a significant reduction in Sino-Nasal Outcome Test 20 (SNOT-20) score with xylitol irrigation as compared to saline irrigation in patients with chronic rhinosinusitis.[114]

Most of the literature on Manuka honey is based on its antimicrobial properties in wound care, such as postoperative infection, burns, nonhealing ulcers, and biofilms in chronic rhinosinusitis secondary to *Staphylococcus aureus* and *Pseudomonas aeruginosa*.[115] The mechanism of action includes acidity, hydrogen peroxide content, osmotic effect, and antioxidant effect and, when ingested, has antibacterial activity by decreasing prostaglandin levels and elevating nitric oxide levels.[116] The use of Manuka honey in sinonasal irrigation for allergic and nonallergic rhinitis needs further assessment.

The use of Dead Sea salt has been found to improve the chronic condition of asthmatics due to its anti-inflammatory and vasodilatatory process. Cordray et al conducted a randomized, single-blind, placebo-controlled study during spring allergy season looking at the treatment of intranasal hypertonic Dead Sea saline spray, triamcinolone spray, and placebo nasal saline spray. This study found a significant reduction in quality of life score in both treatment groups; however, the greatest improvement was seen in the Dead Sea saline group. The dominant cation in the Dead Sea salt is magnesium, which has been shown to be efficacious in treatment of acute asthma by way of relaxing bronchial smooth muscle and influencing inflammatory mediators.[117] When magnesium levels in the blood decrease, eosinophils and histamine levels increase,[118] and magnesium has been shown to prevent eosinophils from undergoing exocytosis and degranulation.[119] Therefore, intranasal hypertonic saline solution may improve symptoms of allergic rhinitis and other symptoms associated with this. Further studies of intranasal Dead Sea salt and the effects on rhinitis are needed.

Other topical intranasal treatments include surfactant, N-chlorotaurine, and sodium hyaluronate. Surfactants, such as 1% baby shampoo and citric acid/zwitterionic surfactant, decrease surface tension and reduce mucus viscosity to facilitate mucociliary clearance.[120] Most studies on the use of surfactants are based on treatment of biofilms in CRS with varied findings and efficacy.[121–123] Further research needs to be done on surfactants and mucociliary clearance in rhinitis. N-chlorotaurine (NCT), a derivative of the amino acid taurine, also has antimicrobial and anti-inflammatory properties that can be applied to the eye, skin ulcerations, and paranasal sinuses.[124] NCT is well tolerated as a nasal irrigation and was found to have benefits in patients with CRS, including decreased mucosal swelling and improved nasal breathing.[125] Sodium hyaluronate is a glycosaminoglycan that is a component of the extracellular matrices and plays a large role in mucociliary clearance. In patients with allergic and nonallergic rhinitis, the combination of intranasal mometasone and sodium hyaluronate was associated with improvement in sneezing, rhinorrhea, and nasal congestion, but not cough, asthma symptoms, or postnasal drip.[126] Therefore, despite its ability to reduce neutrophil count on nasal cytology, further work needs to be done to elucidate the efficacy of sodium hyaluronate on rhinitis.

Capsaicin, the active element of chili peppers, has been used in cough research as a stimulus to induce cough and airway irritation. In chronic cough, capsaicin cough sensitivity is increased and related to cough hypersensitivity. Treatment with topical capsaicin in nonallergic rhinitis has been shown to reduce nasal symptoms and hyperreactivity through the desensitization of cough receptors.[127,128] Capsaicin initially causes irritation to the applied area; however, with multiple uses, the area becomes desensitized, such as areas with nerve endings that cause rhinorrhea, sneezing, and congestion.[129] Yu et al demonstrated that cough sensitivity in UACS was significantly higher than in rhinitis/sinusitis patients without cough and healthy subjects.[62] The proposed hypothesis was that the cough in UACS patients was secondary to sensitization of the C afferents in the upper airway by postnasal drip and inflammation. However, in this study, the nasopharynx was bypassed, and capsaicin was used through an inhaled nebulizer, showing that the sensitization of capsaicin-sensitive cough receptors in the lower airway may be the trigger in cough hypersensitivity. Gerven et al evaluated the mechanism of action of capsaicin in treatment of nonallergic rhinitis and found that capsaicin treatment significantly improved symptoms and nasal hyperreactivity through a decrease in nasal mucosal innervation and downregulation of the TRPV1-SP signaling pathway in the mucosa of the upper and lower airway, of which activation causes neuronal excitation and local inflammatory response.[130] Further studies are needed to shed light on the mechanism of cough hypersensitivity in UACS patients as it relates to lower-airway inflammation.

How Do Nasal Treatments Cure Cough?

Upper airway-directed treatments for chronic cough are primarily targeted toward the primary diagnosis (eg, allergic or nonallergic rhinitis, chronic rhinosinusitis, and UACS). Gawchik et al conducted a randomized, double-blind study to examine the effectiveness of mometasone furoate nasal spray in reducing nasal inflammation in seasonal allergic rhinitis and found there was a significant reduction in daytime cough and nasal symptoms, and nighttime cough to a lesser extent.[92] Therefore, the mechanism of AR-induced cough likely shares the same inflammatory mechanism as those responsible for the nasal symptoms. Consequently, by reducing secretory activity and mucosal inflammation, this also reduces pharyngeal irritability leading to cough.

Treatment strategy should be targeted at the specific diagnosis leading to chronic cough, whether it is predominantly caused by sinonasal disease, lower airway disease, or GERD and LPR from the alimentary tract. The differential diagnosis of cough should be narrowed, and empiric therapy can be trialed prior to further testing and imaging. Reasons for treatment failure include lack of appreciation of all causes for chronic cough,[1] use of empirical trials of therapy with inadequate dose or insufficient duration, and missed diagnosis of primary etiology.

CONCLUSION

In the diagnosis and treatment of chronic cough, both pulmonary and extrapulmonary etiologies need to be considered. Frequently, the cause may be multifactorial and empiric treatment of each disease may ultimately be necessary. The unified airway model draws the connection between the upper and lower airway, and management of both is beneficial in the treatment of chronic cough. Cough-variant asthma, GERD or LPR, and PND, or any combination of these, account for the majority of cough symptoms.[58,59] Therefore, a thorough clinical examination with targeted therapy, in addition to patient education, is the mainstay for successful treatment of chronic cough. Rhinosinogenic etiologies should be considered in the setting of objective evidence of nasal or sinus inflammation by endoscopy and/or imaging. In the absence of these findings, extranasal etiologies should be rapidly incorporated into the differential diagnosis.

THINKING OUTSIDE OF THE BOX

The role of the rhinologist in diagnosis of cough is to provide a thorough evaluation of the upper airway and identify any possible causes. If the medical history and clinical examination identifies an etiology for the cough, appropriate workup, such as with CT, should be completed and the diagnosis treated appropriately. However, because the cause of cough is frequently multifactorial, strong consideration also needs to be given to GERD and LPR as an additional source. If the nasal exam is normal and there are no identifiable causes of cough, GERD and LPR are the culprits until proven otherwise, and empiric therapy is recommended. Successful treatment of chronic cough depends on appropriate dosage and duration of therapy, patient education, and multidisciplinary evaluation.

TAKE-HOME POINTS

- The lower and upper airway are linked through several possible mechanisms and should be thought of within the context of the unified airway.
- The presence and severity of cough and asthma have been epidemiologically associated with upper airway inflammation. By extension, adequate treatment of upper airway inflammation has been shown to have an indirect benefit on the lower airway.

- After exclusion of ACE inhibitor–related or primary lower airway disease, cough variant asthma, GERD/LPR, and UACS account for the vast majority of cough etiologies and can frequently coexist.
- GERD and LPR have been associated with medically refractory chronic rhinosinusitis and failure of endoscopic sinus surgery; therefore, aggressive treatment of reflux is recommended in CRS causes of cough.[44]
- Appropriate workup of the upper airway includes a clinical exam, nasal endoscopy with pharyngoscopy and, when necessary, CT.
- When UACS is suspected, first-line therapies include first-generation antihistamines and intranasal corticosteroids.
- Successful treatment requires selection of the appropriate agent, dose, delivery method, and duration. Patient education and counseling is critical to maximize compliance.

REFERENCES

1. McGarvey LP, Polley L, MacMahon J. Review series: chronic cough: common causes and current guidelines. *Chron Respir Dis.* 2007;4:215–223.
2. Krouse JH, Brown RW, Fineman SM, et al. Asthma and the unified airway. *Otolaryngol Head Neck Surg.* 2007;136(suppl 5):S75–106. doi:10.1016/j.otohns.2007.02.019
3. Meltzer E. The relationships of rhinitis and asthma. *Allergy Asthma Proc.* 2005;26:336–340.
4. Prieto JL, Gutierrez V, Berto JM, Camps B. Sensitivity and maximal response to methacholine in perennial and seasonal allergic rhinitis. *Clin Exp Allergy.* 1996;26:61–67.
5. Seidman MD, Gurgel RK, Lin SY, et al. Clinical practice guideline: allergic rhinitis. *Otolaryngol Neck Surg.* 2015;152:S1–S43.
6. Rosenfeld RM, Andes D, Bhattacharyya N, et al. (2007). Clinical practice guideline: adult sinusitis. *Otolaryngol Head Neck Surg.* 2015;137:S1–S31.
7. Blair H. Natural history of childhood asthma: 20-year follow-up. *Arch Dis Child.* 1977;52:613–619.
8. Smith J. Epidemiology and natural history of asthma, allergic rhinitis and atopic dermatitis (eczema). In: Middleton E, ed., *Allergy: Principles and Practice.* St. Louis, MO: Mosby; 1988:891–929.
9. Pedersen P, Weeke E. Asthma and allergic rhinits in the same patients. *Allergy.* 1983;38:25–29.
10. Settipane G. Allergic rhinitis: update. *Otolaryngol Head Neck Surg.* 1986;94:470–475.
11. Corren J. Allergic rhinitis and asthma: how important is the link? *J Allergy Clin Immunol.* 1997;99(2):S2781–S2786.

12. Broder I, Higgins M, Mathews K, Keller J. Epidemiology of asthma and allergic rhinitis in a total community, Tecumseh, Michigan. *J Allergy Clin Immunol.* 1974;54:100–110.
13. Maternowski C, Mathews K. The prevalence of ragweed pollinosis in foreign and native students at a midwestern university and its implications concerning methods for determining inheritance of atopy. *J Allergy.* 1962;33:130–140.
14. Yawn BP, Yunginger JW, Wollan PC, Reed CE, Silverstein MD, Harris AG. Allergic rhinitis in Rochester, Minnesota residents with asthma: frequency and impact on health care charges. *J Allergy Clin Immunol.* 1999;103(1): 54–59.
15. Krouse JH, Brown RW, Fineman SM, et al. Asthma and the unified airway. *Otolaryngol Head Neck Surg.* 2007;136:S75–S106.
16. Jani A, Hamilos D. Current thinking on the relationship between rhinosinusitis and asthma. *J Asthma.* 2000;106:213–227.
17. Senior BA, Kennedy DW, Tanabodee J, Kroger H, Hassab M, Lanza D. Long-term impact of functional endoscopic sinus surgery on asthma. *Otolaryngol Head Neck Surg.* 1999;12:66–68.
18. Leynaert B, Bousquet J, Neukirch C, Liard R, Neukirch F. Perennial rhinitis: an independent risk factor for asthma in nonatopic subjects: results from the European Community Respiratory Health Survey. *J Allergy Clin Immunol.* 1997;104:301–304.
19. Corren J, Kachru R. Relationship between nonallergic upper airway disease and asthma. *Clin Allergy Immunol.* 2007;19:101–114
20. Louis R, Lau L, Bron A, Roldaan AC, Radermecker M, Djukanović R. The relationship between airways inflammation and asthma severity. *Am J Respir Crit Care Med.* 2000;161:9–16.
21. Robinson D, Hamid Q, Ying S, et al. Predominant TH2-like bronchoalveolar T-lymphocyte population in atopic asthma. *N Engl J Med.* 1992;326(5):298–304.
22. Bradding P, Feather I, Wilson S, et al. Immunolocalization of cytokines in the nasal mucosa of normal and perennial rhinitic subjects. *J Immunol.* 1993;151: 3853–3865.
23. Togias A. Rhinitis and asthma: Evidence for respiratory system integration. *J Allergy Clin Immunol.* 2003;111(6):1171–1183.
24. Halpern M, Schmier J, Richner R, Guo C, Togias A. Allergic rhinitis: a potential cause of increased asthma medication use, costs, and morbidity. *J Asthma.* 2004;41(1):117–126.
25. Pawankar R. Allergic rhinitis and asthma: are they manifestations of one syndrome? *Clin Exp Allergy.* 2006;36:1–4.
26. Committee TECRHSIS. The European Community Respiratory Health Survey II. *Eur Respir J.* 2002;20:1071–1079.
27. Aubier M, Cleriel C, Neukirch F, Herman D. Different effects of nasal and bronchial glucocorticosteroid administration on bronchial hyperresponsiveness in patients with allergic rhinitis. *Am Rev Respir Dis.* 1992;146:122–126.
28. Hirano T, Matsunaga K. Late-onset asthma current perspectives. *J Asthma Allergy.* 2018;11:19–27.
29. Bachert C, Vignola M, Gevaert P, Leynaert B, Van Cauwenberge P, Bousquet J. Allergic rhinitis, rhinosinusitis, and asthma: one airway disease. *Immunol Allergy Clin North Am.* 2004;24:19–43.

30. Dhong H, Hyo K, Cho D. Histopathologic characteristics of chronic sinusitis with bronchial asthma. *Acta Otolaryngol.* 2005;125:169–176.
31. Harlin SL, Ansel DG, Lane SR, Myers J, Kephart GM, Gleich GJ. A clinical and pathologic study of chronic sinusitis: the role of the eosinophil. *J Allergy Clin Immunol.* 1988;81(5 pt 1):867–875.
32. Ponikau JU, Sherris DA, Kephart GM, et al. Features of airway remodeling and eosinophilic inflammation in chronic rhinosinusitis: is the histopathology similar to asthma? *J Allergy Clin Immunol.* 2003;112(5):877–882. doi:10.1016/j.jaci.2003.08.009
33. Bresciani M, Paradis L, Des Roches A, et al. Rhinosinusitis in severe asthma. *J Allergy Clin Immunol.* 2001;107(1):73–80.
34. Ten Brinke A, Grootendorst DC, Schmidt JT, et al. Chronic sinusitis in severe asthma is related to sputum eosinophilia. *J Allergy Clin Immunol.* 2002;109(4):621–626.
35. Bothwell M, Parsons DS, Talbot A, Barbero GJ, Wilder B. Outcome of reflux therapy on pediatric chronic sinusitis. *Otolaryngol Head Neck Surg.* 1999;121:255–262.
36. Phipps C, Wood W, Gibson W, Cochran W. Gastroesophageal reflux contributing to chronic sinus disease in children, a prospective study. *Arch Otolaryngol Head Neck Surg.* 2000;126:831–836.
37. Halstead L. Role of gastroesophageal reflux in pediatric upper airway disorders. *Otolaryngol Head Neck Surg.* 1999;120:208–214.
38. Barbero G. Gatroesophgeal reflux and upper airway disease. *Otolaryngol Clin North Am.* 1996;29:27–38.
39. O'Reilly R, Soundar S, Tonb D, et al. The role of gastric pepsin in the inflammatory cascade of pediatric otitis media. *JAMA Otolaryngol Head Neck Surg.* 2015;141(4):350–357.
40. Leason S, Barham H, Oakley, G, et al. Association of gastro-oesophageal reflux and chronic rhinosinusitis: systematic review and meta-analysis. *Rhinology.* 2017;55(1):3–16.
41. Ulualp S, Toohill R, Hoffmann R, Shaker R. Possible relationship of gastroesophagopharyngeal acid reflux with pathogenesis of chronic sinusitis. *Am J Rhinol.* 1999;13:197–202.
42. DiBiase J, Olusola B, Huerter J, Quigley E. Role of GERD in chronic resistant sinusitis: a prospective, open label, pilot trial. *Am J Gastroenterol.* 2002;97:843–850.
43. DiBiase J, Huerter J, Quigley E. Sinusitis and gastro-esophageal reflux disease. *Ann Intern Med.* 1998;129:1078.
44. DelGaudio J. Direct nasopharyngeal reflux of gastric acid is a contributing factor in refractory chronic rhinosinusitis. *Laryngoscope.* 2005;115:946–957.
45. Chambers D, Davis W, Cook P, Nishioka GJ, Rudman DT. Long-term outcome analysis of functional endoscopic sinus surgery: correlation of symptoms with endoscopic examination findings and potential prognostic factors. *Laryngoscope.* 1997;107:504–510.
46. Kaufman J, Wright G. The effect of nasal and nasopharyngeal irrigation on airway resistance in man. *Am Rev Respir Dis.* 1969;100:626–630.
47. Wyllie J, Kern E, O'Brien P, Hyatt R. Alteration of pulmonary function associated with artificial nasal obstruction. *Surg Forum.* 1976;27:535–537.

48. Nolte D, Berger D. On vagal bronchoconstriction in asthmatic patients by nasal irritation. *Eur J Respir Dis.* 1983;64(suppl):110–114.
49. Madonini E, Briatico-Vangosa G, Pappacoda A, Maccagni G, Cardani A, Saporiti F. Seasonal increase of bronchial reactivity in allergic rhinitis. *J Allergy Clin Immunol.* 1987;79(2):358–363.
50. Ramsdale EH, Morris MM, Roberts RS, Hargreave FE. Asymptomatic bronchial hyperresponsiveness in rhinitis. *J Allergy Clin Immunol.* 1985;75:573–577.
51. Townley R, Ryo U, Kolotkin B, Kang B. Bronchial sensitivity to methacholine in current and former asthmatic and allergic rhinitis and control subjects. *J Allergy Clin Immunol.* 1975;56:429–442.
52. Fontanari P, Burnet H, Zattara-Hartmann M, Jammes Y. Changes in airway resistance induced by nasal inhalation of cold dry, dry, or moist air in normal individuals. *J Appl Physiol.* 1985;81(4):1739–1743.
53. Kaufman J, Chen J, Wright G. The effect of trigeminal resection on reflex bronchoconstriction after nasal and nasopharyngeal irritation in man. *Am Rev Respir Dis.* 1970;101:768–769.
54. Mullen W, Wyder C. Experimental lesions of lungs produced by inhalation of fluid from the nose and throat. *Am Rev Tubere.* 1920;4:683–687.
55. McLaurin J. Chest complications of sinus disease. *Ann Otol Rhinol Laryngol.* 1932;41:780–793.
56. Brugman S, Larsen G, Henson P, Honor J, Irvin C. Increased lower airways responsiveness associated with sinusitis in a rabbit model. *Am Rev Respir Dis.* 1993;147:314–320.
57. Nelson J, Karempelis P, Dunitz J, Hunter R, Boyer H. Pulmonary aspiration of sinus secretions in patients with cystic fibrosis. *Int Forum Allergy Rhinol.* 2018; 8(3):385–388.
58. Pratter M. Overview of common causes of chronic cough. *Chest.* 2006;129:59S–62S.
59. Pratter MR. Chronic upper airway cough syndrome secondary to rhinosinus diseases (previously referred to as postnasal drip syndrome). *Chest.* 2006; 129(1):63S–71S.
60. Pratter MR, Bartter T, Akers S, DuBois J. An algorithmic approach to chronic cough. *Ann Intern Med.* 1993;119:977–983.
61. O'Hara J, Jones N. "Post-nasal drip syndrome": most patients with purulent nasal secretions do not complain of chronic cough. *Rhinology.* 2006;44(4):270–273.
62. Yu L, Xu X, Wang L, Yang Z, Lü H, Qiu Z. Capsaicin-sensitive cough receptors in lower airway are responsible for cough hypersensitivity in patients with upper airway cough syndrome. *Med Sci Monit.* 2013;19:1095–1101. doi:10.12659/MSM.889118
63. Dicpinigaitis P. Effect of viral upper respiratory tract infection on cough reflex sensitivity. *J Thorac Dis.* 2014;6(suppl 7):S708–S711.
64. Tran NP, Vickery J, Blaiss MS. Management of rhinitis: allergic and non-allergic. *Allergy, Asthma Immunol Res.* 2011;3(3):148–156. doi:10.4168/aair.2011.3.3.148
65. Kaliner M. The treatment of vasomotor nonallergic rhinitis. In: Baraniuk J, & Shusterman D, eds. *Nonallergic Rhinitis.* New York, NY: Informa Healthcare USA; 2007:351–362.
66. O'Connell F, Thomas V, Pride N, Fuller R. Capsaicin cough sensitivity decreases with successful treatment of chronic cough. *Am J Respir Crit Care Med.* 1994;150(2):374–380.

67. Song WJ, Morice AH. Cough hypersensitivity syndrome: a few more steps forward. *Allergy, Asthma Immunol Res.* 2017;9(5):394–402.
68. Chung KF, McGarvey L, Mazzone SS. Chronic cough as a neuropathic disorder. *Lancet Respir Med.* 2013;1(5):414–422. doi:10.1016/S2213-2600(13)70043-2
69. Ellegard E, Karlsson N, Ellegard L. Rhinitis in the menstrual cycle, pregnancy, and some endocrine disorders. In: Baraniuk J, Shusterman D, eds. *Nonallergic Rhinitis.* New York, NY: Informa Healthcare USA; 2007: 305–321.
70. Alhussien AH, Alhedaithy RA, Alsaleh SA. Safety of intranasal corticosteroid sprays during pregnancy: an updated review. *Eur Arch Oto-Rhino-Laryngology.* 2017;275(2): 1–9.
71. Unlu H, Akyar S, Caylan R, Nalça Y. Concha bullosa. *J Otolaryngol.* 1994;23: 23–27.
72. Bolger W, Clifford A, Parsons D. Paranasal sinus bony anatomic variations and mucosal abnormalities: CT analysis for endoscopic sinus surgery. *Laryngoscope.* 1991;101:56–64.
73. Cannon C. Endoscopic management of concha bullosa. *Otolaryngol Head Neck Surg.* 1994;110:449–454.
74. Elahi M, Frenklel S, Fageeh N. Paraseptal structural changes and chronic sinus disease in relation to the deviated septum. *J Otolaryngol.* 1997;26:236–240.
75. Alkire BC, Bhattacharyya N. An assessment of sinonasal anatomic variants potentially associated with recurrent acute rhinosinusitis. *Laryngoscope.* 2010; 120(3):631–634.
76. Calhoun K, Waggenspack G, Simpson C, Hokanson J, Bailey B. CT evaluation of the paranasal sinuses in symptomatic and asymptomatic populations. *Otolaryngol Head Neck Surg.* 1991;104(4):480–483.
77. Horwitz Berkun R, Polak D, Shapira L, Eliashar R. Association of dental and maxillary sinus pathologies with ear, nose, and throat symptoms. *Oral Dis.* 2017;July:1–7. doi:10.1111/odi.12805
78. Eloy P, Watelet J, Hatert A, Bertrand B. Thornwaldt's cyst and surgery with powered instrumentation. *B-ENT.* 2006;2(3):135–139.
79. Marzouk H, Aynehchi B, Thakkar P, Abramowitz T, Goldsmith A. The utility of nasopharyngeal culture in the management of chronic adenoiditis. *Int J Pediatr Otorhinolaryngol.* 2012;76(10):1413–1415.
80. Mladina R, Vukovic K, Poje G. The two holes syndrome. *Am J Rhinol Allergy.* 2009;23(6):602–604.
81. Liu H, Sun C, Han Y, Shang G. Analysis of the causes and treatment of postnasal drip syndrome. *Lin Chung Er Bi Yan Hou Tou Jing Wai Ke Za Zhi.* 2008;22(2):68–69.
82. Bartha L, Baumzweiger W, Buscher DS, et al. Multiple chemical sensitivity: a 1999 consensus. *Arch Environ Health,* 1999;54(3):147–149.
83. Rossi S, Pitidis A. Multiple chemical sensitivity: review of the state of the art in epidemiology, diagnosis and future perspectives. *J Occup Environ Med.* 2017; 60(2):138–146.
84. Chung K, Pavord I. Prevalence, pathogenesis, and causes of chronic cough. *Lancet.* 2008;371:1364–1374.
85. Dheda K, Crawford A, Hagan G, Roberts C. Implementation of British thoracic society guidelines for acute exacerbation of chronic obstructive pulmonary disease: impact on quality of life. *Postgr Med J.* 2004;80(941):169–171.

86. Irwin RS, Baumann MH, Bolser DC, et al. Diagnosis and management of cough executive summary: ACCP evidence-based clinical practice guidelines. *Chest.* 2006;129(suppl 1):1S–23S.
87. Hampton T. New guidelines released for managing cough. *J Am Med Assoc.* 2006;295(7):746–747.
88. Editorial. Cough guidelines choke on evidence. *Lancet.* 2006;367(9507):276.
89. Irwin R, Curley F, French C. Chronic cough. The spectrum and frequency of causes, key components of the diagnostic evaluation, and outcome of specific therapy. *Am Rev Respir Dis.* 1990;141(3):640–647.
90. Irwin R, Corrao W, Pratter M. Chronic persistent cough in the adult: the spectrum and frequency of cases and successful outcome of specific therapy. *Am Rev Respir Dis.* 1981;123:413–417.
91. Morice AH, McGarvey L, Pavord I. Recommendations for the management of cough in adults. *Thorax.* 2006;61(suppl 1):1–25.
92. Gawchik S, Goldstein S, Prenner B, John A. Relief of cough and nasal symptoms associated with allergic rhinitis by mometasone furoate nasal spray. *Ann Allergy, Asthma Immunol.* 2003;90(4):416–421.
93. Dicpinigaitis PV, Gayle YE. Effect of the second-generation antihistamine, fexofenadine, on cough reflex sensitivity and pulmonary function. *Br J Clin Pharmacol.* 2003;56(5):501–504.
94. Muether P, Gwaltney J. Variant effect of first- and second-generation antihistamines as clues to their mechanism of action on the sneeze reflex in the common cold. *Clin Infect Dis.* 2001;33:1483–1488.
95. McLeod R, Mingo G, O'Reilly S, Ruck LA, Bolser DC, Hey JA. Antitussive action of antihistamine is independent of sedative and ventilation activity in the guinea pig. *Pharmacology.* 1998;57:57–64.
96. Packman E, Ciccone P, Wilson J, Masurat T. Antitussive effects of diphenhydramine on the citric acid aerosol-induced cough response in humans. *Int J Clin Pharmacol Ther Tox.* 1991;29:218–222.
97. Studham J, Fuller R. The effect of oral terfenadine on the sensitivity of the cough reflex in normal volunteers. *Pulm Pharmacol.* 1992;5:51–52.
98. Tanaka S, Hirata K, Kurihara N, Yoshikawa J, Takeda T. Effect of loratadine, an H1 antihistamine, on induced cough in non-asthmatic patients with chronic cough. *Thorax.* 1996;51:810–814.
99. Lilienfield L, Rose J, Princiotto J. Antitussive activity of diphenhydramine in chronic cough. *Clin Pharmacol Ther.* 1976;19:421–425.
100. Ciprandi G, Buscaglia S, Catrullo A, Marchesi E, Bianchi B, Canonica GW. Loratadine in the treatment of cough associated with allergic rhinoconjunctivitis. *Ann Allergy Asthma Immunol.* 1995;75:115–120.
101. McGarvey L, Heaney L, Lawson J, et al. Evaluation and outcome of patients with chronic non-productive cough using a comprehensive diagnostic protocol. *Thorax.* 1998;53:738–743.
102. Macedo P, Saleh H, Torrego A, et al. Postnasal drip and chronic cough: an open interventional study. *Respir Med.* 2009;103(11):1700–1705.
103. Zanasi A, Lecchi M, Del Forno M, et al. A randomized, placebo-controlled, double-blind trial on the management of post-infective cough by inhaled ipratropium and salbutamol administered in combination. *Pulm Pharmacol Ther.* 2014;29(2):224–232.

104. Holmes P, Barter C, Pierce R. Chronic persistent cough: use of ipratropium bromide in undiagnosed cases following upper respiratory tract infection. *Respir Med.* 1992;86:425–429.
105. Lowry R, Wood A, Higenbottam T. The effect of anticholinergic bronchodilator therapy on cough during upper respiratory tract infections. *Br J Clin Pharmacol.* 1994;37(2):187–191.
106. Dicpinigaitis P, Spinner L, Santhyadka G, Negassa A. Effect of tiotropium on cough reflex sensitivity in acute viral cough. *Lung.* 2008;186:369–374.
107. Bateman ED, Rennard S, Barnes P J, et al. Alternative mechanisms for tiotropium. *Pulm Pharmacol Ther.* 2009;22(6):533–542.
108. Harvey R, Hannan S, Badia L, Scadding G. Nasal saline irrigations for the symptoms of chronic rhinosinusitis. *Cochrane Database Syst Rev, 3.* 2007;CD006394.
109. Van Den Berg J, De Nier L, Kaper N, et al. Limited evidence: higher efficacy of nasal saline irrigation over nasal saline spray in chronic rhinosinusitis–an update and reanalysis of the evidence base. *Otolaryngol Head Neck Surg.* 2014;150:16–21.
110. Pynnonen M, Mukerji S, Kim H, Adams ME, Terrell JE. Nasal saline for chronic sinonasal symptoms: a randomized controlled trial. *Otolaryngol Head Neck Surg.* 2007;133:1115–1120.
111. Brown CL, Graham SM, Cable BB, Ozer EA, Taft PJ, Zabner J. Xylitol enhances bacterial killing in the rabbit maxillary sinus. *Laryngoscope.* 2004;114(11): 2021–2024.
112. Kurola P, Tapiainen T, Sevander J, et al. Effect of xylitol and other carbon sources on STREPTOCOCCUS PNEUMONIAE biofilm formation and gene expression in vitro. *Apmis.* 2011;119(2):135–142.
113. Lin L, Tang X, Wei J, Dai F, Sun G. Xylitol nasal irrigation in the treatment of chronic rhinosinusitis. *Am J Otolaryngol Head Neck Med Surg.* 2017;38(4):383–389. doi:10.1016/j.amjoto.2017.03.006
114. Weissman JD, Fernandez F, Hwang PH. Xylitol nasal irrigation in the management of chronic rhinosinusitis: a pilot study. *Laryngoscope.* 2011;121(11): 2468–2472.
115. Alandejani T, Marsan J, Ferris W, Slinger R, Chan F. Effectiveness of honey on STAPHYLOCOCCUS AUREUS and PSEUDOMONAS AERUGINOSA aeruginosa biofilms. *Otolaryngol Head Neck Surg.* 2009;141(1):114–118.
116. Al-Waili N, Salom K, Butler G, Al Ghamdi A. Honey and microbial infections: a review supporting the use of honey for microbial control. *J Med Food.* 2001; 14(10):1079–1096.
117. Cordray S, Harjo JB, Miner, L. Comparison of intranasal hypertonic Dead Sea saline spray and intranasal aqueous triamcinolone spray in seasonal allergic rhinitis. *Ear, Nose, Throat J.* 2005;84(7):426–430.
118. Chyrek-Borowska S, Obrzut D, Hofman J. The relation between magnesium, blood histamine level and eosinophilia in the acute stage of the allergic reactions in humans. *Arch Immunol Ther Exp.* 1978;26:709–712.
119. Larbi K, Gomperts B. Complex pattern of inhibition by magnesium of exocytosis from permeabilised eosinophils. *Cell Calcium.* 1997;21:213–219.
120. Varshney R, Lee JT. Current trends in topical therapies for chronic rhinosinusitis: update and literature review. *Expert Opin Drug Deliv.* 2017;14(2):257–271.

121. Chiu A, Palmer J, Woodworth B, et al. Baby shampoo nasal irrigations for the symptomatic post-functional endoscopic sinus surgery patient. *Am J Rhinol.* 2008;22:34–37.
122. Farag A, Deal A, McKinney K, et al. Single-blind randomized controlled trial of surfactant vs. hypertonic saline irrigation following endoscopic endonasal surgery. *Int Forum Allergy Rhinol.* 2013;3:276–280.
123. Valentine R, Jervis-Bardy J, Psaltis A, Tan LW, Wormald PJ. Efficacy of using a hydrodebrider and of citric acid/zwitterionic surfactant on a Staphylococcus aureus bacterial biofilm in the sheep model of rhinosinusitis. *Am J Rhinol Allergy.* 2011;25:323–326.
124. Gottardi W, Nagl M. N-chlorotaurine, a natural antiseptic with outstanding tolerability. *J Antimicrob Chemother.* 2010;65(3):399–409.
125. Neher A, Fischer H, Appenroth E. Tolerability of N-chlorotaurine in chronic rhinosinusitis applied via Yamik catheter. *Auris Nasus Larynx.* 2005;32(4):359–364.
126. Gelardi M, Iannuzzi L, Quaranta N. Intranasal sodium hyaluronate on the nasal cytology of patients with allergic and nonallergic rhinitis. *Int Forum Allergy Rhinol.* 2013;3(10):807–813.
127. Ternesten-Hasséus E, Johansson EL, Millqvist E. Cough reduction using capsaicin. *Respir Med.* 2015;109(1):27–37.
128. Lacroix J, Buvelot J, Polla B, Lundberg J. Improvement of symptoms of non-allergic chronic rhinitis by local treatment with capsaicin. *Clin Exp Allergy.* 1991;21:595–600.
129. Kushnir NM. The role of decongestants, cromolyn, guafenesin, saline washes, capsaicin, leukotriene antagonists, and other treatments on rhinitis. *Immunol Allergy Clin North Am.* 2011;31(3):601–617.
130. Van Gerven L, Alpizar YA, Wouters MM, et al. Capsaicin treatment reduces nasal hyperreactivity and transient receptor potential cation channel subfamily V, receptor 1 (TRPV1) overexpression in patients with idiopathic rhinitis. *J Allergy Clin Immunol.* 2014;133(5).

4

REFLUX DISEASE

Matthew P. Partain and Jonathan M. Bock

INTRODUCTION

Gastroesophageal reflux (GER) and laryngopharyngeal reflux (LPR) are both common diagnoses associated with the development of airway irritation and inflammation. GER is a term that refers to the retrograde transit of gastric contents into the esophagus, occurring with or without regurgitation into the pharynx or vomiting. LPR is defined as the retrograde flow of gastric contents into the laryngopharynx, leading to irritation and inflammation of the upper aerodigestive tract.[1] Symptoms associated with LPR are generally nonspecific and can include such varied presentations as chronic cough, dysphonia, throat clearing, subglottic stenosis, and globus sensation. Clinical instruments commonly used to evaluate LPR include the Reflux Finding Score (RFS) and the Reflux Symptom Index (RSI).[2–4] Unfortunately, these instruments have generally been found to be neither sensitive nor specific for determining Gastroesophageal Reflux Disease (GERD) related to chronic cough. Refluxate consists of hydrochloric acid, gastric pepsin, bacteria, bile salts, and pancreatic digestive enzymes, all of which may have effects on the esophageal and airway mucosa. Episodes of reflux can occur up to 50 times a day, usually during meals and the postprandial state in healthy individuals, and may be entirely asymptomatic in the majority of patients.[5] Reflux is commonly indicated as a potential cause for chronic cough, but these associations can often be hard to prove without a thorough evaluation. Direct correlation or causation of pathologic GER or LPR with development of classic LPR symptoms can therefore be challenging to prove.

GERD refers to a disease process caused by GER and manifested by symptoms and physical cellular tissue damage.[6] These symptoms include postprandial heartburn, supine reflux, choking spells at night, regurgitation, taste of acid in the mouth, heartburn, halitosis, retrosternal chest pain, vomiting, and tooth enamel degradation.[7] GER-related symptoms such as heartburn, regurgitation, and dysphagia are incredibly common, and were found to be present in almost 60% of patients in a recent population-based study.[8] It is also critically important to remember that the diagnosis of GERD alone does not establish a causal relationship between reflux and chronic cough. The establishment of a GERD-related cause of cough requires at least some assessment of the temporal relationship between reflux episodes and cough bursts.[9] LPR, however, may not always have direct symptom correlation with reflux events and a cough as has been shown in post-antireflux surgery patients diagnosed with the newest impedance technology.

PREVALENCE OF GERD AS A CAUSE OF COUGH

Cough represents a complex protective reflex that requires an elegant coordination of sensory input, respiratory function, and muscle action in response to noxious stimuli. When looking broadly at causes of chronic cough in patients referred to otolaryngologists, postnasal drip, asthma, and GERD were the cause of cough in 86% of patients. This increased to 99.4% of patients when considering those who were immunocompetent nonsmokers who were also not on ACE inhibitor therapy.[10] It is certainly appropriate and worthwhile to have a pulmonologist evaluate the patient for intrinsic lung pathology such as asthma, COPD, and nonasthmatic eosinophilic bronchitis prior to considering GERD as the sole cause of the patient's chronic cough.[11,12] In 2016, the journal *Chest* released updated chronic cough care guidelines and an expert panel report that proposed a clinical profile for a patient with chronic cough that was likely due to GER even without concomitant GI symptoms.[13] There is no question that GERD and LPR have been overly diagnosed as the primary etiology for challenging cough cases over the last 20 years. Studies have shown that most patients with unexplained chronic cough tested for reflux with dual pH impedance testing do not actually demonstrate pathologic proximal or distal reflux events on dual pH impedance testing.[1] This, however, may be called into question as more research is done using impedance catheters that traverse the upper esophageal sphincter and as pathologic hypopharyngeal reflux events are more well defined.

While a small number of patients may present with silent nonacid reflux as a cause of chronic cough, several studies have shown that the vast majority of patients with reflux-related chronic cough are more likely to present with classic heartburn symptoms. Patients with heartburn are also more likely to respond to proton-pump inhibitor medications for treatment, prompting the latest revisions in the 2016 *Chest* cough guidelines recommending against empiric PPI trials for cough patients.[13] It is therefore our opinion, based on the currently available data, that reflux is a relatively rare but important cause of chronic cough symptomatology. That being the case, the most difficult cases of refractory cough can be due to undiagnosed nonacid reflux, and when patients present to quaternary referral centers, this should be thoroughly evaluated. This is discussed in detail in Chapter 9.

MECHANISMS OF COUGH STIMULATION BY REFLUX

The cough reflex is a complicated mechanism under voluntary and involuntary control mediated by C fibers and pulmonary stretch muscles of the tracheobronchial tree. More recently, afferent vagal fibers innervating the esophagus and upper aerodigestive tract have been shown to be present and involved in the cough reflex. There is a convergence of these vagal afferents at sites of brainstem integration at the nucleus tractus solitarius of the medulla, which has been shown to be intimately involved in the cough reflex.[14,15] GERD can stimulate the afferent limb of the cough reflex by irritating the upper aerodigestive tract and larynx with gastric contents. Microaspiration or macroaspiration can also irritate the lower respiratory tract, leading to chronic recurrent coughing episodes.[16] There is also strong evidence to support that acid in the esophagus alone is enough to stimulate an esophageal-tracheobronchial cough reflex. A study by Harding et al found episodic chronic cough to have a temporal relationship with acid exposure in the distal esophagus and not proximal aid exposure.[10] Ninety percent of patients with GERD-related cough had coughing within 5 minutes of a reflux event seen on a pH probe placed at the lower esophageal sphincter. Thus, even gastric refluxate into the distal esophagus alone can lead to a sufficient stimulus to trigger a coughing event, and this is in fact a relatively common mechanism for GERD-related chronic cough in symptomatic patients. Coughing alone can also induce GER episodes through increased intra-abdominal pressure, and a cough-GER self-perpetuating cycle may be involved in the pathophysiology of a patient's chronic cough.[17]

DIAGNOSIS OF REFLUX

Clinical Presentation and Initial Evaluation

GERD-related cough is difficult to clinically characterize, as cough presentation can be incredibly variable.[18] Most patients with cough related to reflux have a dry, nonproductive cough. Patients with comorbid pulmonary disease such as bronchiectasis or chronic bronchitis may conversely present with mixed or even frankly productive cough, and having these comorbidities does not rule out the contribution of LPR. A general evaluation of cough is appropriate prior to consideration of reflux as a cause. This evaluation should include the following:[19]

- Current or heavy prior tobacco use may obviate further testing for cause aside from appropriate pulmonary consultation and evaluation.
- Medications that can cause cough such as angiotensin-converting enzyme inhibitors and angiotensin receptor blockers should be held for a trial period.
- Chest x-ray or computed tomography (CT) should be performed in all patients with cough for more than 4 weeks. Low-dose lung cancer screening CT may also be considered for appropriate patients.
- Common pulmonary causes of cough such as cough-variant asthma or nonasthmatic eosinophilic bronchitis should be ruled out with pulmonary function testing with methacholine challenge, sputum studies, and possible bronchoscopy with bronchoalveolar lavage. Many authors would further suggest a trial of several weeks of inhaled corticosteroid.
- Allergies and sinusitis have been properly evaluated and trials of appropriate medications have been performed to rule out upper airway cough syndrome (UACS).

Patients with pathologic reflux may be clinically "silent" up to 75% of the time, meaning overt GERD-related symptoms may be absent. Many of these patients may have esophageal hypersensitivity with referred laryngeal irritation. However, chronic cough due to reflux should always be considered seriously with concurrent GERD-related symptoms of frequent heartburn and regurgitation.

ENDOSCOPY

Endoscopic evaluation of the larynx has traditionally been used to examine for the standard laryngeal harbingers of LPR. These include edema of the supraglottic structures and pharyngeal walls, posterior laryngeal pachydermia ("piled up" interarytenoid mucosa), diffuse laryngeal erythema, ventricular obliteration, laryngeal pseudosulcus (a linear furrow in the anteroposterior plane of the true vocal fold that appears due to inferior true vocal fold swelling and is not a true scar/sulcus vocalis), and thickened laryngeal secretions. It is imperative that physicians not assume inflammatory laryngeal changes are specific solely to GERD. These findings are associative at best, and are generalized signs of laryngeal inflammation that could be from many potential other sources including obstructive sleep apnea, laryngeal allergy, or even systemic diseases such as sarcoidosis or amyloidosis.[20]

The initial diagnostic test of choice for GER evaluation from the gastroenterology perspective is traditionally esophagogastroduodenoscopy (EGD) with biopsy to evaluate for inflammation or dysplasia. Patients with reflux esophagitis often will present with endoscopic and/or histopathologic changes indicative of ongoing esophageal mucosal injury and inflammation. The presence of these typical findings of reflux esophagitis on EGD may have a specificity as high as 97%. EGD can unfortunately be negative in up to 50% of patients with reflux symptoms, with findings therefore suggestive of nonerosive reflux disease.[21] Severity of GERD symptom presentation correlates poorly with the degree of underlying esophageal damage on EGD biopsies, likely due to the ability of the esophageal mucosa to tolerate insult and heal rapidly once injured. Many patients with significant LPR/GERD-related symptoms may in fact suffer from esophageal motility disorders and may benefit from further testing with high-resolution manometry (HRM). HRM can detect altered esophageal peristalsis, esophageal sphincter incompetence, and neurologic injury, and may further be combined with esophageal impedance to detect bolus passage and regurgitation.

Laryngeal endoscopy and videostroboscopy facilitate the detection of other causes of dysphonia, globus, or throat clearing due to glottic insufficiency and should be performed on all patients with chronic cough to rule out other organic sources of laryngeal irritation. Most recent research in the field of LPR has used survey-based instruments to establish an LPR clinical diagnosis, a process that is uncertain at best. Patient-based survey instruments such as the RSI and endoscopic reflux severity indexes such as the RFS are fraught with deep variability due to the vague nature of traditional LPR patient complaints and the overlap of these symptoms with other possibly confounding conditions.[22] The RFS in particular is often used in clinical practice by the general otolaryngology community to infer reflux-related damage to the laryngopharynx by the potential association of reflux with laryngeal edema, erythema, and thickened secretions. Studies have shown that laryngeal endoscopy may be suggestive of ongoing reflux but is far from a certain association due to the myriad other causes of these nonspecific laryngeal findings.

OBJECTIVE REFLUX TESTING

This intrinsic challenge in establishing an appropriate diagnosis for the patient with suspected LPR on endoscopy alone often necessitates further objective testing in many patients, particularly when symptoms are severe or surgical intervention is being considered. There is no single standardized approach to objective reflux testing in clinical practice. Several testing options are currently utilized in the otolaryngology and gastroenterology communities, each with specific benefits and controversies for evaluation of chronic cough. We feel strongly that objective reflux testing for the patient with suspected LPR should include proximal esophageal and pharyngeal impedance data if possible. Many patients can demonstrate physiologic distal esophageal reflux but have extensive proximal excursion of reflux boluses, which would be overlooked with testing modalities that only evaluate distal esophageal reflux. Multichannel intraluminal impedance with dual pH (MII-pH) probe testing provides the most useful data in this regard in our estimation. MII-pH probes include dual pH sensors located in the distal esophagus and proximal esophagus or hypopharynx, depending on probe selection and placement. These probes also include paired impedance arrays straddling the distal pH sensor and a third set in the proximal esophagus, which allows for detection of anterograde and retrograde bolus transit. New impedance/pH probes have specifically been designed for use in the LPR patient to assess proximal acid and nonacid reflux in this regard, such as the ComforTec LPR probe array (Diversatek, Milwaukee, WI, USA). The term HEMII-pH probes will be used to describe the LPR probes due to the hypopharyngeal-esophageal multichannel intraluminal impedance and dual pH nature of the catheter. This term is used and referenced later in this book (see Chapter 9). These studies allow for determination of a DeMeester score for evaluation of traditional GERD, and facilitate the study of symptom association with both distal and proximal reflux events. There continues to be significant controversy in the interpretation of proximal esophageal impedance data in the literature due to varying probe array utilization and placement, but most studies support that frequent proximal esophageal and hypopharyngeal reflux events are abnormal in healthy adult patients.[23,24]

The standard approach to LPR evaluation in the gastroenterology clinic is via EGD and placement of a single distal esophageal wireless capsule-based sensor for pH evaluation (such as the Bravo reflux testing system, Medtronic, Minneapolis, MN, USA). These wireless systems are well tolerated by the patient, and provide excellent data for evaluation of traditional GERD, including calculation of a DeMeester score. Current recommendations from the gastroenterology literature support the use of these ambulatory pH testing systems for all patients with classic GERD. They do not, however, provide any information regarding nonacid reflux and do not measure proximal extent of reflux. We have found that many patients may demonstrate normal distal reflux but have abnormal proximal migration of refluxate, much of which may be nonacid and therefore missed by wireless capsule testing.

Temporal symptom association correlations between coughing spells and reflux episodes can be very helpful in assessing reflux-related cough pathology. A recent blinded, cross-sectional study by Francis et al used concurrent time-synchronized audio and MII-pH to measure reflux events and phonation triggers in patients with idiopathic chronic cough.[25] They found that the probability of cough increased with higher burdens of reflux. Also of note was that antecedent pH-impedance events were immediately found to be associated with an increased rate of de novo cough, and this was statistically significant. Seventy percent of patients with chronic cough exhibited a temporal relationship between reflux and cough.

The gastric digestive enzyme pepsin has been shown to be a reliable molecular marker for the diagnosis of reflux.[26] It is solely produced by chief cells located in the gastric mucosa and, therefore, all refluxate, both nonacidic and acidic, has pepsin as a constituent. Pepsin has further been shown to be a causative agent of laryngeal damage and inflammation in acidic and nonacidic reflux, as it can be activated by acidic dietary elements once deposited in the pharynx and larynx. Pepsin found within laryngeal tissues and oropharyngeal secretions may therefore link LPR with GERD. Ongoing studies are attempting to delineate a causal relationship between pepsin presence in the endolarynx and symptoms of LPR.[27] Recently, in a small prospective study, seven of eight adults experienced improvement in symptoms such as heartburn and cough, as well as elimination of pepsin from laryngeal biopsies after antireflux surgery.[28] A molecular marker such as pepsin would be of great use. See Chapter 5 for further information on the current state of pepsin testing in the management of cough.

TREATMENT

Diet and Lifestyle Management

Diet and lifestyle changes have been shown in prior studies to be effective in reducing reflux, and may have an impact on chronic cough issues due to this. Weight loss in general has a beneficial effect on reflex, as increased abdominal fat increases basal intra-abdominal pressure and risk of obstructive sleep apnea and reflux events. Randomized, controlled trials of weight loss in severely obese individuals have documented decreases in esophageal reflux with lowered body mass index. Weight loss is challenging for most patients, however, and maintaining weight loss long term is even harder. Other general lifestyle recommendations may also include suggestions to quit smoking, decrease caffeine consumption, and limit use of carbonated beverages, as these have all been shown to reduce GERD symptoms. Specific low-fat, low-acid, and antireflux diets have recently become popular among many patients, and are of low risk but have little data to support beneficial outcomes. Chocolate, red wine, and mint have also been shown to decrease lower esophageal sphincter tone and may increase reflux. Elevating the head of the bed even 3 to 4 inches above the foot (extra pillows, including a wedge, are often ineffective due to the patient sliding down to a flat position during sleep) also reduces the frequency and strength of reflux episodes due to the effect of gravity, as can sleeping in left lateral decubitus position. Certain medications have also been shown to increase esophageal reflux, such as aspirin, nitrates, and calcium channel blockers.[2]

Medication Trials

Patients with chronic cough who have symptoms consistent with GERD (such as heartburn, regurgitation, or pyrosis) should be evaluated for reflux as a primary intervention after pulmonary causes of cough are ruled out. This may include EGD with biopsies, barium esophagram if solid food dysphagia is present, and/or empiric medication trials. If significant GERD symptoms are present without dysphagia warning signs (odynophagia, weight loss, food impaction, hematemesis), no further testing is necessarily required before the option of starting a trial of medical antireflux therapy after visualization of the larynx. Maximum medication trials for GERD include using a proton-pump inhibitor (PPI) twice daily, taken 30 minutes before breakfast and dinner for 2 to 3 months.[30] Clinicians may also consider addition of an adjunct therapy of nighttime H2 blocker. Prokinetics such as metoclopramide are generally reserved for treatment of GERD in children.[31] Adherence to a medication trial is important as PPI therapy may not be effective if taken in intermittent fashion.[27] Sodium alginate suspensions (such as those present in Gaviscon Advance from the UK) may also be of use for patients with nonacid reflux or inability to take PPI medication due to allergy or medical contraindications. These medications are thought to prevent liquid regurgitation through the lower esophageal sphincter by resting on top of gastric contents as a physical barrier, and have been shown in some studies to decrease GERD and LPR symptoms.[32] Alginates must be taken four or more times throughout the day (typically after meals and at bedtime) as they are digested and gone when the stomach empties. It is crucial that the clinician follow up with the patient, preferably 3 months after a medication trial is initiated, to assess response to treatment. If successful, the patient may be able to be slowly weaned off medication. Further objective reflux testing, preferably HEMII-pH testing if available, is often indicated if the patient does not respond despite a strong supportive history of possible ongoing reflux.[33]

ANTIREFLUX SURGERY

Surgical intervention is traditionally used to treat the more typical reflux symptoms such as heartburn, regurgitation, and severe hiatal hernia, but it may also be of significant value in the management of reflux-related cough. Studies relating to outcomes of surgical treatment of GERD often suffer from lack of controls and blinding, and different preoperative/postoperative evaluation criteria. Kaufman and colleagues reported their long-term outcomes of 128 patients treated with laparoscopic antireflux surgery. Cough and hoarseness was improved in 65% to 75% of cases, compared to heartburn and regurgitation in more than 90% of patients.[34] A study by Jobe et al also demonstrated significant improvement in cough symptoms in carefully selected patients with increased proximal reflux following fundoplication, with 13 out of 16 patients showing total resolution.[35] Another review of treatment options for GERD-related cough summarized the findings of nine prospective studies of surgical management, reporting that 85% of surgically treated patients had a "significant cough response."[36] Studies have continued to show that many patients with reflux-related cough have normal DeMeester scores and significant nonacid reflux burden, suggesting that HEMII-pH testing may be necessary to truly evaluate these patients for possible surgical intervention.[37]

Further testing is required by many gastric surgeons to document the extent of reflux prior to referral for surgical consultation. This testing can include upper endoscopy of the aerodigestive tract, barium esophagram, esophageal manometry, and formal pH probe testing (MII-pH, HEMI-pH, or wireless capsule). It is generally recommended that the following indicators be met:[38,39]

- 24-hour ambulatory pH monitoring study is positive (either dual pH-MII, HEMII-pH, or distal esophageal wireless pH system).
- Patient symptom profile fits diagnosis of GERD, and other obvious causes of cough have been adequately ruled out as described above.
- Lack of response to medical regimen or failure to tolerate medication.
- Ongoing sequelae of GERD (esophagitis, Barrett's esophagus, hiatal hernia).
- Adequate esophageal motility present to allow for fundoplication and avoid postoperative dysphagia.
- Cough severity is sufficient to impede patient quality of life (and in these cases, with patient understanding risks of surgery, typical GERD complaints such as known heartburn and regurgitation may not be required before proceeding).[40,41]

Nissen fundoplication is a time-tested surgical treatment modality for patients with refractory reflux, and studies have published outcome data for more than 20 years. Studies have consistently shown that carefully selected patients may benefit from fundoplication procedures to improve chronic cough, globus, dysphonia, and other LPR-related symptoms with proper patient selection.[42,43] Cough patients have generally been shown to have the best improvement if they had pre-existing heartburn and traditional GERD symptoms. The Linx Reflux Management System is designed to augment the LES through magnetomechanical means.[7] It utilizes a circular ring of magnetic beads that are designed to resist expansion mimicking the native LES. This does impact the ability for a patient to undergo an MRI though the newer versions of the system are compatible with 1.5 tesla MRIs. Laparoscopic Rou-en-Y gastric bypass has been demonstrated as the most effective bariatric surgical procedure for the improvement of symptoms related to GERD for obese patients. Qualifications beyond the previously mentioned surgical referral criteria include patients with BMI >40 or >35 with two or more obesity-related comorbidities such as type II diabetes, hypertension, obstructive sleep apnea, heart disease, or lipid abnormalities, among others. Long-term evidence shows improvement in patients with GERD who undergo surgical intervention, justifying early referral for surgical evaluation when patients meet criteria.[7,28]

CONCLUSIONS

Management of a patient with reflux-related chronic cough requires astute clinical evaluation and the use of objective data. This begins with careful history taking and evaluation of other potential and more common causes of cough, including thorough pulmonary evaluation. Patients with wet productive cough, ongoing tobacco use history, ACE inhibitor use, and abnormal chest imaging are not likely to have reflux-related chronic cough. Further testing for reflux-related cough in properly selected patients may include empiric PPI trials and/or ambulatory objective reflux testing depending on patient and treating center preference. Close follow-up examination and discussion of symptom improvement or persistence is crucial in the management of patients with suspected reflux-related chronic cough. Research continues to evolve regarding the association between gastric enzymes such as pepsin and its role in LPR and symptoms such as chronic cough, as well as normative data for proximal esophageal and hypopharyngeal impedance. It is crucial to document the presence of abnormal esophageal acid exposure when antireflux surgery is to be considered, and we vastly prefer HEMII-pH testing with proximal hypopharyngeal impedance and pH to truly assess the extent of nonacid reflux in symptom presentation. The results of objective testing help to establish the presence of abnormal esophageal reflux and assist with intensity of treatment through careful cost and benefit analysis of medical versus surgical intervention. Additional randomized studies with long-term follow-up are required to evaluate the diagnostic and therapeutic benefit of new technologies such as HEMII-pH and pepsin testing.

THINKING OUTSIDE OF THE BOX: CHRONIC COUGH AND REFLUX

Chronic cough due to reflux is a rare creature, and it is unfortunate that many patients have been misdiagnosed in this regard in the PPI era of modern medicine. The vast majority of patients seen in our tertiary laryngology referral clinic for cough evaluation have nonreflux causes, especially non-acidic reflux casuses, for cough. The majority have cough due to pulmonary issues, sinusitis, ACE inhibitor use, or glottic insufficiency. Many patients with reflux are asymptomatic, and many patients with cough related to reflux may not have abnormal proximal reflux and simply suffer from esophageal hypersensitivity. The clinician must use a careful treatment algorithm to properly select cough patients for reflux evaluation and potential treatment. It is also crucial that cough patients have adequate follow-up with their care team to establish outcomes of diagnostic testing, response to treatment, and discussion of ongoing care and potential weaning off medications. Many patients are placed on PPI medication for trial periods and stay on them for decades without clear reasoning. We also feel strongly that speech pathologist evaluation and treatment can be highly beneficial for all patients with chronic cough to decrease cough severity and alleviate behavioral contributions to chronic laryngeal irritation (see Chapter 8).

The traditional gastroenterology evaluation of patients with atypical symptoms of GERD, including chronic cough, includes EGD with distal wireless ambulatory pH probe testing. The gastroenterology community has waned in enthusiasm for MII-pH testing over the last several years due to the variability of normative data and the lack of supportive long-term follow-up studies showing benefit of surgical intervention based on predictive impedance-based symptom association protocols. Data from our group and others are slowly building to support the role for MII-pH, specifically HEMII-pH, evaluation to detect those patients with normal DeMeester scores and non-GERD presentations who still have elevated proximal reflux events with concomitant symptomology. Many patients with normal total reflux (measured by percentage of time under pH 4.0) with persistent full-column or hypopharyngeal reflux are missed with these traditional evaluation methods. Further data are needed to establish useful normative data and pathologic data for both proximal esophageal and hypopharyngeal acid and nonacid reflux; this will require more surgical outcome data for patients selected for antireflux surgery based on objective reflux testing parameters. To date, most studies have included small numbers of patients with promising results, but variability in testing methods, probe selection, and data interpretation have made a broad consensus challenging for the true establishment of reliable normative values.

TAKE-HOME POINTS

- Chronic cough due to reflux is well described but is still a challenging clinical diagnosis to establish in some patients.
- Rule out other much more common causes of cough prior to reflux testing and/or empiric medication trials. These more common causes include concomitant tobacco use, pulmonary causes, UACS/sinusitis, and ACE inhibitor use.
- Lifestyle and dietary recommendations, including encouraging tobacco cessation and weight loss, should be considered for all patients when appropriate.
- Offer patients early objective reflux testing using MII-pH and, if available, HEMII-pH, to expedite proper diagnosis. Although standard distal esophageal capsule pH testing can evaluate for traditional GERD, many patients with atypical GERD (ie, LPR) symptoms will have normal total amounts of reflux with elevated proximal extent making these testing modalities of little use.
- If an empiric trial of PPI is pursued as initial treatment, clinical follow-up in 2 to 3 months is crucial to evaluate treatment response and provide ongoing treatment planning. Indefinite treatments for PPI medications is often unnecessary and should be monitored.
- Surgical referral for consideration of fundoplication or gastric bypass may be appropriate for many patients with elevated DeMeester score, hiatal hernia, or morbid obesity, as well as for rarer patients without these findings but with intractable chronic cough in the face of known high esophageal and pharyngeal reflux events.

- Further prospective research on normative proximal esophageal and hypopharyngeal impedance data, biologic reflux markers such as pepsin, and novel surgical technique outcomes for patients with reflux and chronic cough is sorely needed.

REFERENCES

1. Cumpston EC, Blumin JH, Bock JM. Dual pH with multichannel intraluminal impedance testing in the evaluation of subjective laryngopharyngeal reflux symptoms. *Otolaryngol Head Neck Surg.* 2016;155(6):1014–1020. doi:10.1177/0194599816665819
2. Belafsky P, Postma G, Koufman J. The validity and reliability of the reflux finding score (RFS). *Laryngoscope.* 2001;111(8):1313–1317. doi:10.1097/00005537-2001080000-00001
3. Ford CN. Evaluation and management of laryngopharyngeal reflux. *JAMA.* 2005;294(12):1534. doi:10.1001/jama.294.12.1534
4. Chen M, Hou C, Chen T, Lin Z, Wang X, Zeng Y. Reflux symptom index and reflux finding score in 91 asymptomatic volunteers. *Acta Oto-Laryngol.* 2018;138(7):659–663. doi:10.1080/00016489.2018.1436768
5. Irwin RS. Chronic cough due to gastroesophageal reflux disease. *Chest.* 2006;129(1). doi:10.1378/chest.129.1_suppl.80s
6. Johnston N, Dettmar PW, Strugala V, Allen JE, Chan WW. Laryngopharyngeal reflux and GERD. *Ann N Y Acad Sci.* 2013;1300(1):71–79. doi:10.1111/nyas.12237
7. Kethman W, Hawn M. New approaches to gastroesophageal reflux disease. *J Gastrointest Surg.* 2017;21(9):1544–1552. doi:10.1007/s11605-017-3439-5
8. Locke G, Talley N, Fett S, Zinsmeister A, Melton L. Prevalence and clinical spectrum of gastroesophageal reflux: a population-based study in Olmsted County, Minnesota. *Gastroenterol.* 1997;112(5):1448–1456. doi:10.1016/s0016-5085(97)70025-8
9. Morice A. Recommendations for the management of cough in adults. *Thorax.* 2006;61(suppl 1):i1–i24. doi:10.1136/thx.2006.065144
10. Harding SM, Richter JE. The role of gastroesophageal reflux in chronic cough and asthma. *Chest.* 1997;111(5):1389–1402. doi:10.1378/chest.111.5.1389
11. Martin MJ, Harrison TW. Causes of chronic productive cough: An approach to management. *Resp Med.* 2015;109(9):1105–1113. doi:10.1016/j.rmed.2015.05.020
12. Cockcroft D. Eosinophilic bronchitis as a cause of cough. *Chest.* 2000;118(1):277. doi:10.1378/chest.118.1.277
13. Kahrilas PJ, Field SK, Harding SM, et al; CHEST Expert Cough Panel. Chronic cough due to gastroesophageal reflux in adults: Chest Guideline and Expert Panel report. *Chest.* 2016;150(6):1341–1360. doi:10.1016/j.chest.2016.08.1458
14. Chung K. Review series: chronic cough: future directions in chronic cough: mechanisms and antitussives. *Chron Respir Dis,* 2007;4(3):159–165. doi:10.1177/1479972307077894
15. Herregods TVK, Pauwels A, Jafari J, et al. Determinants of reflux-induced chronic cough. *Gut.* 2017;66(12):2057–2062. doi:10.1136/gutjnl-2017-313721

16. Decalmer S, Stovold R, Houghton LA, et al. Chronic cough: relationship between microaspiration, gastroesophageal reflux and cough frequency. *Chest.* 2012;142(4):958–964. doi:10.1378/chest.12-0044
17. Francis DO, Slaughter JC, Ates F, et al. Airway hypersensitivity, reflux, and phonation contribute to chronic cough. *Clin Gastroenterol Hepatol.* 2016;14(3):378–384. doi:10.1016/j.cgh.2015.10.009
18. Harding SM, Richter JE. The role of gastroesophageal reflux in chronic cough and asthma. *Chest.* 1997;111(5):1389–1402. doi:10.1378/chest.111.5.1389
19. Irwin RS. Chronic cough due to gastroesophageal reflux disease. *Chest.* 2006; 129(1). doi:10.1378/chest.129.1_suppl.80s
20. ASGE Standards of Practice Committee; Muthusamy VR, Lightdale JR, Acosta RD, et al. The role of endoscopy in the management of GERD. *Gastrointest Endosc.* 2015;81(6):1305–1310. doi:10.1016/j.gie.2015.02.021
21. Badillo R. Diagnosis and treatment of gastroesophageal reflux disease. *World J Gastrointest Pharmacol Ther.* 2014;5(3):105. doi:10.4292/wjgpt.v5.i3.105
22. Chang B, MacNeil S, Morrison M, Lee P. The reliability of the reflux finding score among general otolaryngologists. *J Voice.* 2015;29(5):572–577. doi:10.1016/j.jvoice.2014.10.009
23. Zerbib F, Roman S, Bruley Des Varannes S, et al; Groupe Français De Neuro-Gastroentérologie. Normal values of pharyngeal and esophageal 24-hour pH impedance in individuals on and off therapy and interobserver reproducibility. *Clin Gastroenterol Hepatol.* 2013;11(4):366–372. doi:10.1016/j.cgh.2012.10.041
24. Hoppo T, Sanz AF, Nason KS, et al. How much pharyngeal exposure is "normal"? normative data for laryngopharyngeal reflux events using hypopharyngeal multichannel intraluminal impedance (HMII). *J Gastrointest Surg.* 2011;16(1):16–25. doi:10.1007/s11605-011-1741-1
25. Francis DO, Slaughter JC, Ates F, et al. Airway hypersensitivity, reflux, and phonation contribute to chronic cough. *Clin Gastroenterol Hepatol.* 2016;14(3):378–384. doi:10.1016/j.cgh.2015.10.009
26. Rosen R, Johnston N, Hart K, Khatwa U, Nurko S. The presence of pepsin in the lung and its relationship to pathologic gastro-esophageal reflux. *Neurogastroenterol Motil.* 2011;24(2). doi:10.1111/j.1365-2982.2011.01826.x
27. Samuels TL, Johnston N. Pepsin as a marker of extraesophageal reflux. *Ann Otol Rhinol Laryngol.* 2010;119(3):203–208. doi:10.1177/000348941011900310
28. Wassenaar E, Johnston N, Merati A, et al. Pepsin detection in patients with laryngopharyngeal reflux before and after fundoplication. *Surg Endosc.* 2011; 25(12):3870–3876. doi:10.1007/s00464-011-1813-z
29. Ness-Jensen E, Hveem K, El-Serag H, Lagergren J. Lifestyle intervention in gastroesophageal reflux disease. *Clin Gastroenterol Hepatol.* 2016;14(2). doi:10.1016/j.cgh.2015.04.176
30. Kahrilas PJ, Howden CW, Hughes N, Molloy-Bland M. Response of chronic cough to acid-suppressive therapy in patients with gastroesophageal reflux disease. *Chest.* 2013;143(3):605–612. doi:10.1378/chest.12-1788
31. Chang AB, Lasserson TJ, Gaffney J, Connor FL, Garske LA. Gastro-oesophageal reflux treatment for prolonged non-specific cough in children and adults. *Cochrane Database Syst Rev.* 2011;(1):CD004823.
32. Reimer C, Lødrup A, Smith G, Wilkinson J, Bytzer P. Randomised clinical trial: alginate (Gaviscon Advance) vs. placebo as add-on therapy in reflux patients

with inadequate response to a once daily proton pump inhibitor. *Aliment Pharmacol Ther.* 2016;43(8):899–909. doi:10.1111/apt.13567
33. Irwin RS, French CT. Cough and gastroesophageal reflux: identifying cough and assessing the efficacy of cough-modifying agents. *Am J Med.* 2011;111(8):45–50. doi:10.1016/s0002-9343(01)00820-8
34. Kaufman JA, Houghland JE, Quiroga E, Cahill M, Pellegrini CA, Oelschlager BK. Long-term outcomes of laparoscopic antireflux surgery for gastroesophageal reflux disease (GERD)-related airway disorder. *Surg Endosc.* 2006;20(12):1824–1830. doi:10.1007/s00464-005-0329-9
35. Hoppo T, Komatsu Y, Jobe BA. Antireflux surgery in patients with chronic cough and abnormal proximal exposure as measured by hypopharyngeal multichannel intraluminal impedance. *JAMA Surg.* 2013;148(7):608. doi:10.1001/jamasurg.2013.1376
36. Chandra KD, Harding SM. Therapy insight: treatment of gastroesophageal reflux in adults with chronic cough. *Nat Clin Pract Gastroenterol Hepatol.* 2007;4(11):604–613. doi:10.1038/ncpgasthep0955
37. Suzuki T, Seki Y, Okamoto Y, Hoppo T. Hypopharyngeal multichannel intraluminal impedance leads to the promising outcome of antireflux surgery in Japanese population with laryngopharyngeal reflux symptoms. *Surg Endosc.* 2017;32(5):2409–2419. doi:10.1007/s00464-017-5940-z
38. Fisichella P, Patti M. GERD procedures: when and what? *J Gastrointest Surg.* 2014;18(11):2047-2053. doi:10.1007/s11605-014-2558-5
39. Jobe BA, Richter JE, Hoppo T, et al. Preoperative diagnostic workup before antireflux surgery: an evidence and experience-based consensus of the esophageal diagnostic advisory panel. *J Am Coll Surg.* 2013;217(4):586–597. doi:10.1016/j.jamcollsurg.2013.05.023
40. Altman KW, Irwin RS. Cough: a new frontier in otolaryngology. *Otolaryngol Head Neck Surg.* 2011;144(3):348–352. doi:10.1177/0194599810396136
41. French CL, Irwin RS, Curley FJ, Krikorian CJ. Impact of chronic cough on quality of life. *Arch Intern Med.* 1998;158(15):1657. doi:10.1001/archinte.158.15.1657
42. Hoppo T, Komatsu Y, Jobe BA. Antireflux surgery in patients with chronic cough and abnormal proximal exposure as measured by hypopharyngeal multichannel intraluminal impedance. *JAMA Surg.* 2013;148(7):608. doi:10.1001/jamasurg.2013.1376
43. Carroll TL, Nahikian K, Asban A, Wiener D. Nissen fundoplication for laryngopharyngeal reflux after patient selection using dual pH, full column impedance testing. *Ann Otol Rhinol Laryngol.* 2016;125(9):722–728. doi:10.1177/0003489416649974

5

BASIC SCIENCE CONSIDERATIONS FOR LARYNGOPHARYNGEAL REFLUX (LPR)

Miles Klimara and Nikki Johnston

INTRODUCTION

Laryngopharyngeal reflux (LPR) is considered one of several common causes of chronic cough. Although acidic contents of gastric refluxate have traditionally been viewed as a predominating factor in the etiology of reflux-mediated disease, other components present in gastric reflux such as the enzyme pepsin are increasingly viewed as both biomarkers for and potential mediators of the underlying pathophysiology. In particular, mounting evidence points to the ability of pepsin to incite a proinflammatory response in esophageal and laryngeal epithelium, even in the context of weakly acidic or nonacid reflux, perhaps explaining the observed inefficacy of proton-pump inhibitor (PPI) therapy in the treatment of LPR and chronic cough in the absence of classic symptoms of gastroesophageal reflux disease (GERD). To this end, pepsin inhibition is an important target for drug discovery programs, which may lead to the creation of novel therapies that could address nonacid components of reflux-mediated disease.

BIOMARKERS IN REFLUX AND CHRONIC COUGH

LPR is known as one of several potential etiologies of chronic cough. However, there are limited and mixed data to support both the reliability and specificity of current tools designed to assist in diagnosis of chronic cough and LPR, which range from symptom inventories to laryngoscopic grading schemes.[1–4] As such, there has been considerable investigation into the utility of various biomarkers as predictors of LPR-associated chronic cough. In particular, pepsin is produced exclusively by the chief cells of the stomach, and hence its presence outside of the stomach has been posited as a sensitive biomarker for reflux and aspiration of gastric contents.[5] In intubated pediatric patients, the sensitivity and specificity of pepsin in bronchoalveolar lavage (BAL) samples for predicting clinically identified aspiration have been found to be up to 80% and up to 100%, respectively.[6] Moreover, pepsin has been detected in significantly elevated levels in BAL and tracheal lavage samples acquired from patients with proximal esophageal reflux and chronic cough symptoms, suggesting that BAL pepsin may be a useful measure in differentiating chronic cough secondary to esophageal reflux as opposed to other etiologies.[6,7]

Previous literature has supported pepsin in induced sputum as a potential tool for identifying the presence of proximal refluxate (75% sensitive, 91% specific), which may enter the laryngopharynx and contribute to laryngeal hyperresponsiveness and pulmonary disease.[8] Given the invasiveness of BAL collection, this represents a compelling potential target, and indeed, several studies, discussed below, have compared the utility of pepsin in salivary and induced sputum samples in the detection of LPR to previously validated methods such as the reflux symptom index (RSI, questionnaire useful in determining the severity of reflux-attributed upper respiratory symptoms),[4] reflux finding score (RFS, a tool for grading of laryngoscopic findings indicative of reflux-attributed inflammation),[3] and multichannel intraluminal impedance-pH (MII-pH) monitoring, with impedance spanning the esophagus and hypopharynx widely considered ideal for proximal reflux monitoring.

In patients with chronic upper respiratory symptoms indicative of laryngeal hyperresponsiveness—such as chronic cough, globus sensation, dyspnea, and episodic choking—Spyridoulias et al found a specificity of 0.78 for the presence of salivary pepsin as a predictor for inflammatory changes on laryngoscopy, but a sensitivity of only 0.53.[9] Notably, pepsin did not significantly correlate with reflux symptom inventory scores or reflux events on MII-pH monitoring, and many patients had discordant results between various testing modalities.[9] However, almost half of patients with pulmonary symptoms but minimal inflammatory changes on laryngoscopy had detectable salivary pepsin, perhaps suggesting that mild LPR may be sufficient to cause symptoms of laryngopharyngeal hyperresponsiveness without inducing any visible changes in the airway.[9]

The utility of pepsin as a biomarker for LPR in adult populations with chronic cough without history of symptoms concerning for gastroesophageal reflux appears less promising. In an unselected group of chronic cough patients, induced sputum pepsin has been found to be inversely related to cough frequency, and furthermore these patients do not have significant amounts of proximal reflux by MII-pH.[10] This is suggestive of the notion that in contrast to cough in the setting of LPR, chronic cough secondary to other etiologies may in fact be protective in facilitating the clearance of refluxate and hence preventing microaspiration. These results are consistent with prior studies on pepsin in tracheal lavage specimens, which have found tracheal lavage pepsin to have poor predictive value in an unselected population of patients with chronic respiratory symptoms, but much more sensitive and specific when specifically restricting its use to patients with the aforementioned classic symptoms. Moreover, this may be interpreted as suggestive that LPR is not a major mediator in the pathology of a patient with chronic cough who does not also manifest classic symptoms of GERD, and that in the absence of classical GERD symptoms, evaluation for biochemical evidence of LPR is likely to have limited utility. In stark contrast, others have argued that LPR is in fact the primary etiology of most chronic cough via induction of hyperresponsiveness of the upper airway to noxious stimulation,[11] which, if true, would imply that current methods used for detection of pepsin simply do not accurately reflect the underlying reflux events. Additionally, recent studies using hypopharyngeal-esophageal MII with dual pH (HEMII-pH) to diagnose LPR in patients with chronic cough demonstrated that carefully selected patients have a complete or partial response to Nissen fundoplication despite lack of symptom correlation to cough.[12] This further supports the theory that nonacid LPR may be a chronic underlying inflammatory condition secondary to pepsin deposition in the laryngopharynx and/or esophagus, on top of which other factors trigger the cough, not necessarily a coordinated reflux event.

The lipid-laden alveolar macrophage index (LLMI), similarly, has been suggested as a marker for aspiration of gastric refluxate as it reflects endocytosis of refluxed food lipids by macrophages in bronchoalveolar lavage specimens. Staining of cells within the BAL fluid with oil red O reveals the lipids that can be quantified with the LLMI, which, in prior studies, has been demonstrated to be up to 100% sensitive but only 57% specific for pulmonary aspiration.[13] However, this measure likely has poor utility for investigating chronic cough, as LLMI is not significantly elevated in children with GERD or chronic cough.[6] It has been suggested that the LLMI may reflect endocytosis not only of food lipids, but also of lipids from degradation of alveolar phospholipids,[6] which may account for its poor specificity. As such, although the LLMI may have some limited value in evaluation of aspiration related disease, its utility in the setting of chronic cough is likely very low.

Numerous challenges exist in the development of a biomarker for use as a diagnostic tool in reflux-associated pulmonary disease. The sensitivity and specificity of salivary pepsin are not sufficient to be considered a highly reliable test in isolation, and collection of samples at only a single time point has been suggested to result in false negatives in patients who are not actively refluxing.[9] Therefore, at this time, salivary and BAL pepsin represent one potential tool to aid in the differential diagnosis of chronic pulmonary complaints consistent with laryngeal hyperresponsiveness, and salivary pepsin is particularly appealing, as it does not require specialized equipment or cause patient discomfort. LLMI offers relatively greater sensitivity at the cost of poor specificity, and of course requires the acquisition of BAL specimens, which is prohibitive in many clinical contexts.

PEPSIN AS A MEDIATOR OF INFLAMMATORY DISEASE PROCESSES

In vitro studies have shown that via receptor-mediated endocytosis, nonacid pepsin can enter the epithelium of the hypopharynx and larynx.[14,15] Following endocytosis, receptors and ligands are sorted within weakly acidic late endosomes and the transreticular Golgi (TRG), raising the possibility of pepsin transport via these pathways. Immunoelectron microscopic findings have supported this notion, having identified colocalization of pepsin with the late endosome marker Rab-9 and the TRG marker TRG-46.[16] The TRG has a weakly acidic pH of approximately 5, at which pepsin has roughly 40% of its maximal activity[17,18]; as such, inactive pepsin might potentially be taken up by laryngeal epithelial cells and be activated within intracellular compartments of low pH, setting the stage for intracellular damage (Figure 5–1). Downstream, exposure of hypopharyngeal cells to pepsin at pH 7 has been shown to induce the expression of several proinflammatory cytokines and receptors, including IL-1α, the neutrophil chemoattractant IL-8, and the eosinophil colony-stimulating factor IL-5.[19] Conversely, exposure of laryngeal epithelium to pepsin has been shown to deplete protective proteins such as Sep70 and carbonic anhydrase-III, implying multiple pathways by which pepsin-mediated cell damage might contribute to ongoing inflammation and the endoscopic findings of LPR disease.[18] Moreover, the aforementioned proinflammatory cytokine profile, induced in hypoharyngeal tissues independent of acidic refluxate, is similar to that expressed in reflux esophagitis and is known to contribute to ongoing inflammation in the pathophysiology of GERD.[19]

The above research identifies a novel mechanism by which pepsin might induce cellular injury and inflammation irrespective of the acidity of the extracellular environment, potentially proffering an explanation for the persistence of chronic mucosal inflammation, symptoms, and endoscopic

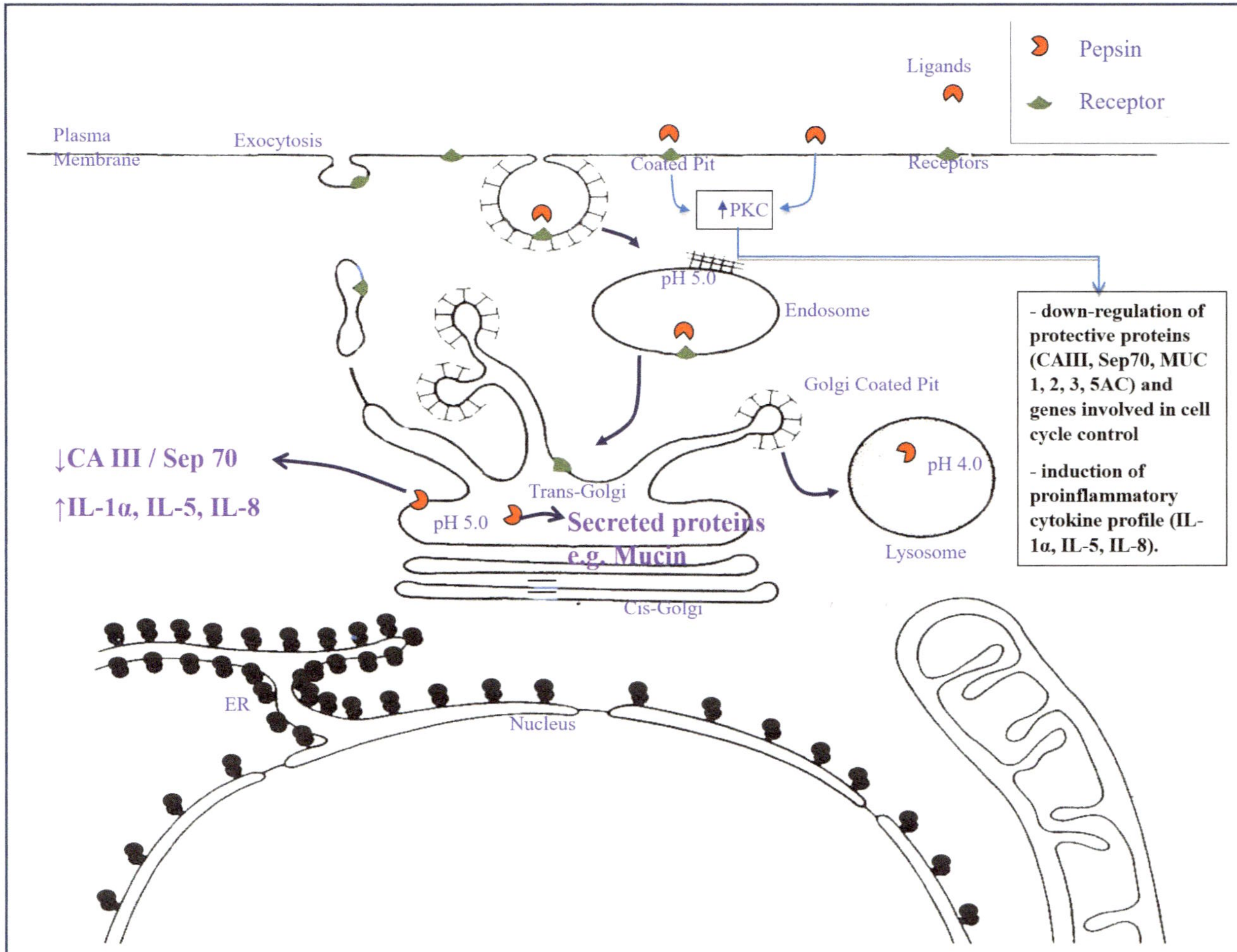

Figure 5–1. Receptors and their ligands are typically sorted in late endosomes and the TRG. When inactive pepsin is taken up by laryngeal epithelial cells by receptor-mediated endocytosis, it may be reactivated in these intracellular compartments of lower pH and thereby cause intracellular damage. Alternatively, binding/activation of the cell surface receptor may induce a cell-signaling event that negatively affects cell function.

findings in many patients with reflux-attributed laryngeal pathology in spite of therapy with high-dose acid suppression. While pepsin has long been known to play an etiologic role in GERD due to its proteolytic activity in the low-pH environment induced by gastroesophageal reflux episodes, the finding of potentially active intracellular pepsin and induction of a proinflammatory response suggests a role for pepsin in reflux-mediated disease of the airway where pH may be less clinically relevant. The receptor mediated uptake of nonacid pepsin, as can occur following LPR, and any inflammatory or neoplastic changes that may occur as a result,[11,19–21] cannot be prevented by PPIs, which only address acid production in gastric mucosa. As the role of pepsin in LPR-mediated mucosal damage seems to involve its activation within more acidic intracellular compartments or through dysregulation or activation of cell-signaling cascades,[16] the amelioration of the acidic environment of gastric refluxate with PPI or histamine (H_2 receptor) antagonists may not adequately address pepsin-mediated inflammatory changes.

Although PPIs remain the mainstay for treatment of GERD, there is poor evidence for their efficacy in the treatment of airway reflux-mediated disease, including LPR.[22] It is widely believed that the upper airway is more sensitive to reflux than the esophagus, and therefore higher dose PPIs are necessary for the control of LPR-related symptoms.[23–25] At this time, placebo-controlled studies by and large have not shown a significant therapeutic benefit to PPIs used in LPR.[26–31] Although some studies have noted evidence of symptomatic improvement with PPI therapy,[32,33] upon review of these two studies, it has been argued that the affected patients only had significant improvement of gastroesophageal reflux symptoms rather than improvement of upper airway symptoms.[30] Arguments can be made that these studies were done prior to the era of HEMII-pH testing, and that the diagnosis of nonacid reflux was incomplete. In light of the poor data for the efficacy of acid suppression in treatment of extraesophageal reflux, the American Gastroenterological Association has specifically recommended against the empiric use of PPIs for suspected LPR unless there are concomitant symptoms of GERD.[34] Likely as a result of the paucity of alternative effective therapies, however, PPIs continue to be used for LPR,[35] and indeed the American Academy of Otolaryngology—Head and Neck Surgery has recommended empiric use of high-dose PPI therapy for suspected LPR, with laparoscopic fundoplication proposed as an alternative to medical management.[24] A recent survey from the American Bronchoesophagological Association reported that twice-daily PPIs remain a popular first-line therapy for LPR.[36]

Laparoscopic fundoplication and magnetic ring procedures are well-established, reliable options for the surgical management of GERD. In contrast to the predictable improvement seen in the treatment of GERD, research on the efficacy of antireflux surgery in the treatment of LPR is mixed, with various studies showing resolution of chronic cough ranging from 63% up to 85% of patients.[37–39] Hypotheses for this variance range from differences in surgical technique to differences in patient selection criteria. In particular, it has been observed that patients with more severe stereotypical GERD symptoms are more likely to benefit from antireflux surgery,[37,40] and in particular patients with preoperative heartburn and pH <4 for more than 12% of a 24-hour period have been found to have a 90% probability of symptomatic improvement.[40]

The role of nonacid reflux in LPR is additionally supported by findings using MII-pH monitoring, which represents a major advance in the diagnosis of extraesophageal reflux disease due to its ability to detect nonacidic reflux events. MII-pH has demonstrated a strong association of LPR symptoms,[41] which, combined with the previously described research revealing poor evidence for the efficacy of acid suppression in LPR and the substantial improvement of symptomatology following surgical intervention such as fundoplication that prevents refluxate from reaching the laryngopharynx,[12,40,42,43] suggests the nonacid components of refluxate must play a major role in the pathophysiology of laryngopharyngeal reflux with chronic cough. In the absence of clear consensus or guidelines regarding the appropriateness of antireflux surgery, preoperative evaluation of esophageal reflux events and motility with MII-pH and high-resolution esophageal manometry has been suggested as a useful tool in predicting postoperative symptom improvement.[12,43] These smaller studies refute the claim that GERD alone predicts response to Nissen by utilizing the newest HEMII-pH technology to select candidates for ant-reflux surgery.[12,43]

Prior in vitro studies have also suggested that bile can cause laryngeal inflammation irrespective of pH, but others have countered that no evidence exists for this as a mechanism of injury to the human larynx.[44] While in vitro exposure to bile acids causes "blebbing" of cell membranes,[45] to our knowledge there are no reports of this histologic finding in laryngeal mucosa of patients with LPR. Notably, previous studies have used high concentrations of bile salts and acids, ranging from 5 to 50 mM. This overlaps the physiologic concentration of bile salts in the human duodenum, which ranges from 10 to 22 mM.[46] In contrast, the physiological bile acid/salt content in gastric refluxate reaching the laryngopharynx is expected to be in the micromolar range,[47] which to our knowledge has not been known to cause damage to laryngeal mucosa. Further, unconjugated bile acids, which cause damage at higher pH such as that of the laryngopharynx, are rarely found as components of gastric refluxate.[11,47] However, there is no strong evidence for the concentration of each bile acid within the laryngopharynx, and the role of bile acids in the pathophysiology of LPR thus remains a dilemma. As such, the previous prevailing understanding of LPR and airway reflux as acid-mediated disease have shifted to a model in which disease is largely mediated by nonacid components of refluxate in which traditional medical management with acid suppression is not sufficient.[48]

PEPSIN AS A THERAPEUTIC TARGET

As discussed above, PPIs continue to be commonly used in clinical practice for the treatment of airway reflux disease including LPR in spite of poor evidence for their efficacy,[26–31] with approximately $26 billion spent yearly for this indication.[49] In light of the inefficacy of PPI therapy for LPR and its associated costs and potential risks, there is substantial interest in an alternative modality for the treatment of LPR.[48,50,51]

Pepsin represents an exciting potential novel target for future therapies, particularly for patients who experience symptoms refractory to PPI therapy in light of its role in nonacid LPR.[16,48] Prior literature has identified two mechanisms by which pepsin might be targeted in therapy of LPR: by irreversible inactivation and via receptor antagonism.[16,48] While the first of these would prevent pepsin's reactivation within the acidic environment of intracellular compartments (Figure 5–2A), the latter would prevent its endocytosis and perhaps the previously described induction of expression of a proinflammatory cytokine profile (Figure 5–2B). Although Pepstatin A is a potent inhibitor of pepsin activity and is currently commercially available, its poor pharmacokinetics and water-soluble characteristics make it a relatively poor candidate for the purpose of treating LPR. As such, novel agents targeting pepsin are currently in development and represent an exciting potential avenue for the treatment of reflux-mediated disease including LPR and chronic cough.

THINKING OUTSIDE OF THE BOX

Although the above literature identifies a clear role for pepsin in the pathophysiology of LPR and chronic cough, studies investigating the utility of salivary pepsin as a marker of extraesophageal reflux found mixed results. Although this may suggest pepsin is not a useful biomarker for airway disease, it is important to remember that salivary levels of pepsin may only be transiently elevated as a result of the transient nature of reflux and intermittent influence of swallowing, both of which will vary with food intake. To that end, optimization of the timing and method of acquisition of salivary samples to yield the greatest balance of sensitivity and specificity is essential if pepsin is to be used clinically as a marker of disease. Although salivary and sputum samples are typically collected at least 1 hour after meals to avoid detection of postprandial reflux events, there have not been any large-scale studies to determine the optimal timing or method of sample collection, and hence the optimal timing for collection of samples is still unclear. Larger studies with more frequent collection of samples may allow

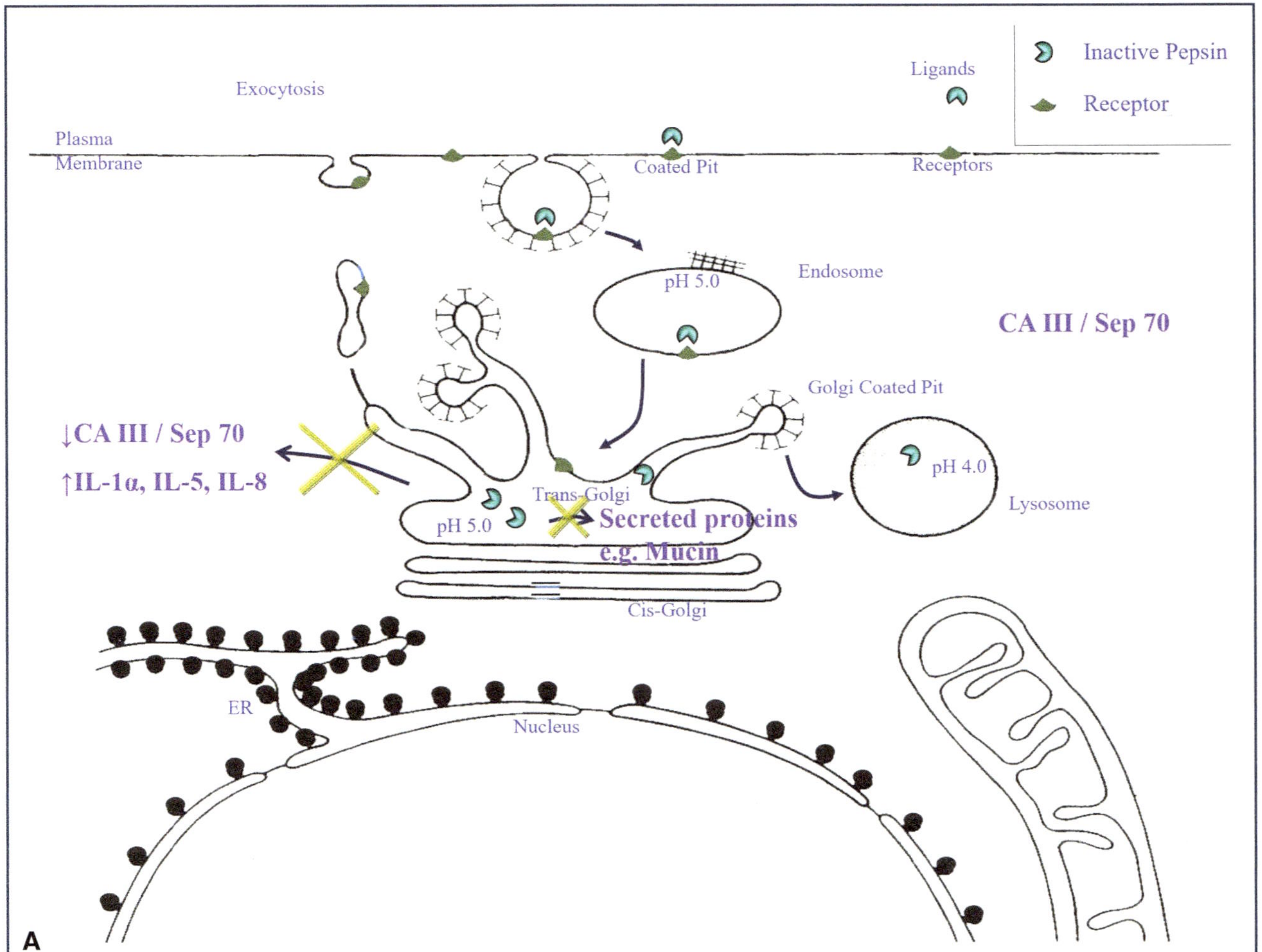

Figure 5–2. A. An irreversible inhibitor of pepsin would prevent inactive pepsin taken up by laryngeal epithelial cells from becoming reactivated in intracellular compartments of lower pH. *continues*

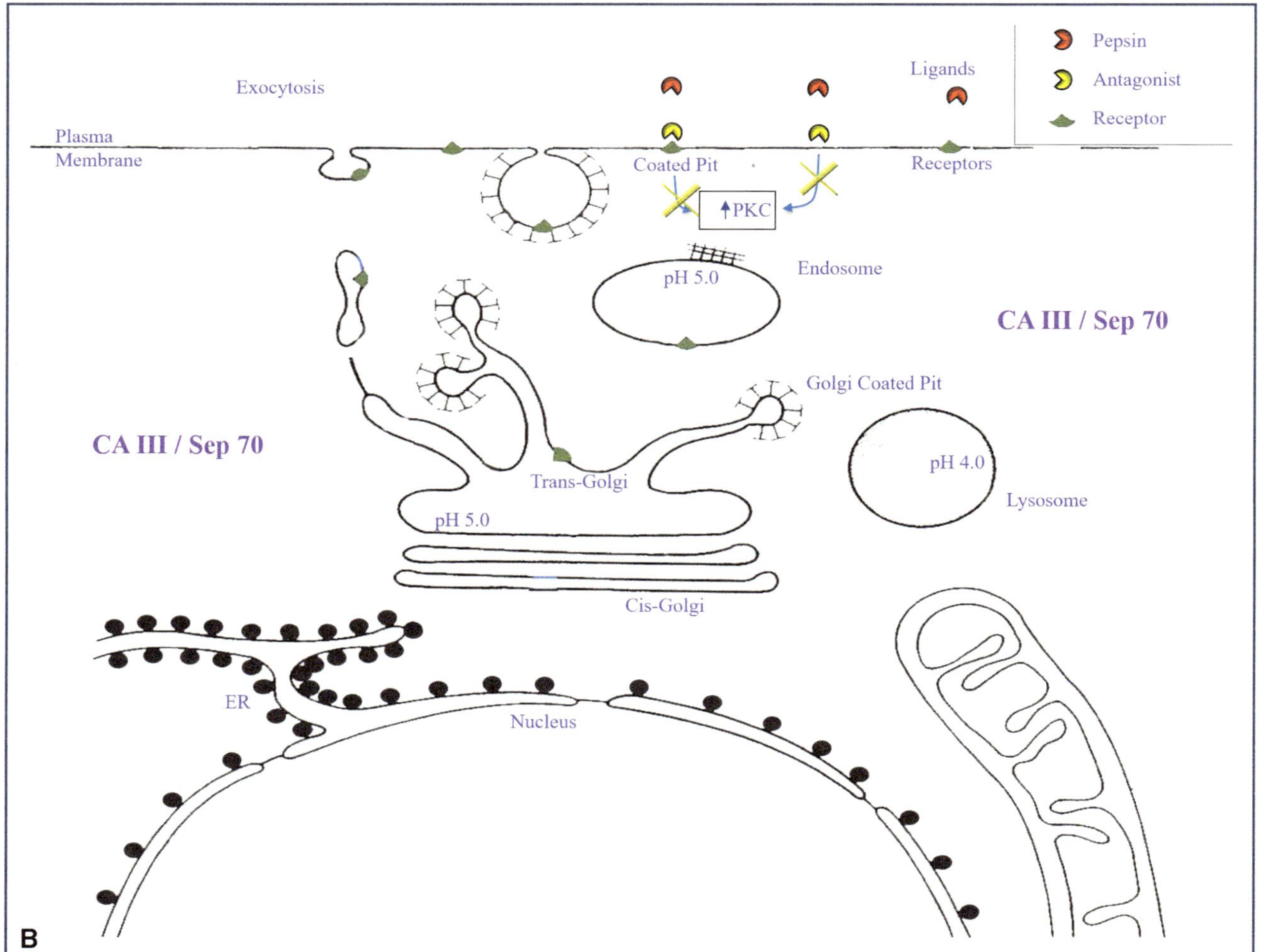

Figure 5–2. *continued*
B. A specific pepsin receptor antagonist would prevent peptic injury via inhibition of its uptake and downstream modulation of cell signaling.

determination of the ideal time for sample collection, which might in turn facilitate the use of salivary pepsin as a more sensitive and specific tool for diagnosing airway disease. Furthermore, salivary pepsin may help to identify a specific subset of chronic cough patients whose reflux and aspiration contributes to their disease, and thus a subset of patients who might benefit from lifestyle modifications for reflux and surgery.

While salivary pepsin does represent evidence of reflux events, and tracheal or BAL pepsin is clear evidence of aspiration, measurement of pepsin in secretions may not adequately reflect its uptake via receptor-mediated endocytosis in laryngeal and lung epithelial cells. As such, intracellular pepsin and tissue-bound pepsin may be more indicative of pepsin-mediated disease than salivary or tracheal/BAL pepsin. Other factors, such as compromise of mucosal defense mechanisms of the tissues in question, may predispose to increased endocytosis of pepsin, setting the stage for its intracellular activation and downstream development of an inflammatory response. Although the invasiveness of sample collection would likely preclude the use of pepsin within tissues as a diagnostic marker, the precise role of pepsin in LPR and chronic cough may be elucidated by future studies examining both factors, which might contribute to increased receptor-mediated endocytosis of pepsin and the relationship between pepsin in salivary secretions and pepsin in laryngeal tissues.

TAKE-HOME POINTS

- The gastric enzyme pepsin is a biochemical marker of reflux-mediated disease that may have utility in understanding LPR and chronic cough.
- Evidence for the utility of biochemical markers in the diagnosis or management of chronic cough associated with LPR is insufficient to recommend their use in clinical practice.
- At this time, careful history and tools including MII-pH (preferably with impedance spanning the esophagus and hypopharynx, HEMII-pH), laryngoscopy, and bronchoscopy are more likely to prove fruitful in establishing the etiology of chronic cough symptoms.
- In light of the poor efficacy of PPIs for reflux-associated chronic cough in patients who lack traditional GERD symptoms (eg, heartburn), nonacid components of refluxate are likely important mediators of the underlying pathophysiology and targets for future research.

- While the role of antireflux surgery in treating LPR and chronic cough is unclear at this time, its potential utility in spite of the poor efficacy of PPIs is similarly suggestive of the role played by nonacid components of refluxate.
- Although pepsin has traditionally been thought to be capable of inducing inflammation only in an acidic environment, there is compelling evidence that nonacid pepsin can cause damage to tissues even at a more neutral pH.
- Pepsin inhibitors and receptor antagonists represent targets for development of novel therapies for reflux-related disease that is refractory to PPI therapy.

REFERENCES

1. Joniau S, Bradshaw A, Esterman A, Carney AS. Reflux and laryngitis: a systematic review. *Otolaryngol Head Neck Surg.* 2007;136(5):686–692.
2. Chang BA, MacNeil SD, Morrison MD, Lee PK. The reliability of the reflux finding score among general otolaryngologists. *J Voice.* 2015;29(5):572–577.
3. Belafsky PC, Postma GN, Koufman JA. The validity and reliability of the reflux finding score (RFS). *Laryngoscope.* 2001;111(8):1313–1317.
4. Belafsky PC, Postma GN, Koufman JA. Validity and reliability of the reflux symptom index (RSI). *J Voice.* 2002;16(2):274–277.
5. Samuels TL, Johnston N. Pepsin as a marker of extraesophageal reflux. *Ann Otol Rhinol Laryngol.* 2010;119(3):203–208.
6. Farrell S, McMaster C, Gibson D, Shields, MD, McCallion WA. Pepsin in bronchoalveolar lavage fluid: a specific and sensitive method of diagnosing gastro-oesophageal reflux-related pulmonary aspiration. *J Pediatr Surg.* 2006; 41(2):289–293.
7. Rosen R, Johnston N, Hart K, Khatwa U, Nurko S. The presence of pepsin in the lung and its relationship to pathologic gastro-esophageal reflux. *Neurogastroenterol Motil.* 2012;24(2):129–133, e184-125.
8. Potluri S, Friedenberg F, Parkman HP, et al. Comparison of a salivary/sputum pepsin assay with 24-hour esophageal pH monitoring for detection of gastric reflux into the proximal esophagus, oropharynx, and lung. *Dig Dis Sci.* 2003; 48(9):1813–1817.
9. Spyridoulias A, Lillie S, Vyas A, Fowler SJ. Detecting laryngopharyngeal reflux in patients with upper airways symptoms: symptoms, signs or salivary pepsin? *Respir Med.* 2015;109(8):963–969.
10. Decalmer S, Stovold R, Houghton LA, et al. Chronic cough: relationship between microaspiration, gastroesophageal reflux, and cough frequency. *Chest.* 2012;142(4):958–964.
11. Pearson JP, Parikh S, Orlando RC, et al. Review article: reflux and its consequences—the laryngeal, pulmonary and oesophageal manifestations. Conference held in conjunction with the 9th International Symposium on Human

Pepsin (ISHP) Kingston-upon-Hull, UK, 21–23 April 2010. *Aliment Pharmacol Ther.* 2011;33(suppl 1):1–71.
12. Suzuki T, Seki Y, Okamoto Y, Hoppo T. Hypopharyngeal multichannel intraluminal impedance leads to the promising outcome of antireflux surgery in Japanese population with laryngopharyngeal reflux symptoms. *Surg Endosc.* 2017;32(5):2409–2419.
13. Corwin RW, Irwin RS. The lipid-laden alveolar macrophage as a marker of aspiration in parenchymal lung disease. *Am Rev Respir Dis.* 1985;132(3):576–581.
14. Johnston N, Wells CW, Samuels TL, Blumin JH. Pepsin in nonacidic refluxate can damage hypopharyngeal epithelial cells. *Ann Otol Rhinol Laryngol.* 2009;118(9): 677–685.
15. Johnston N, Wells CW, Blumin JH, Toohill RJ, Merati AL. Receptor-mediated uptake of pepsin by laryngeal epithelial cells. *Ann Otol Rhinol Laryngol.* 2007; 116(12):934–938.
16. Johnston N, Wells CW, Samuels TL, Blumin JH. Rationale for targeting pepsin in the treatment of reflux disease. *Ann Otol Rhinol Laryngol.* 2010;119(8):547–558.
17. Piper DW, Fenton BH. pH stability and activity curves of pepsin with special reference to their clinical importance. *Gut.* 1965;6(5):506–508.
18. Johnston N, Dettmar PW, Bishwokarma B, Lively MO, Koufman JA. Activity/stability of human pepsin: implications for reflux attributed laryngeal disease. *Laryngoscope.* 2007;117(6):1036–1039.
19. Samuels TL, Johnston N. Pepsin as a causal agent of inflammation during nonacidic reflux. *Otolaryngol Head Neck Surg.* 2009;141(5):559–563.
20. Johnston N, Yan JC, Hoekzema CR, et al. Pepsin promotes proliferation of laryngeal and pharyngeal epithelial cells. *Laryngoscope.* 2012;122(6):1317–1325.
21. Kelly EA, Samuels TL, Johnston N. Chronic pepsin exposure promotes anchorage-independent growth and migration of a hypopharyngeal squamous cell line. *Otolaryngol Head Neck Surg.* 2014;150(4):618–624.
22. Martinucci I, de Bortoli N, Savarino E, et al. Optimal treatment of laryngopharyngeal reflux disease. *Ther Adv Chronic Dis.* 2013;4(6):287–301.
23. Ford CN. Evaluation and management of laryngopharyngeal reflux. *JAMA.* 2005;294(12):1534–1540.
24. Koufman JA, Aviv JE, Casiano RR, Shaw GY. Laryngopharyngeal reflux: position statement of the committee on speech, voice, and swallowing disorders of the American Academy of Otolaryngology-Head and Neck Surgery. *Otolaryngol Head Neck Surg.* 2002;127(1):32–35.
25. Park W, Hicks DM, Khandwala F, et al. Laryngopharyngeal reflux: prospective cohort study evaluating optimal dose of proton-pump inhibitor therapy and pretherapy predictors of response. *Laryngoscope.* 2005;115(7):1230–1238.
26. Eherer AJ, Habermann W, Hammer HF, Kiesler K, Friedrich G, Krejs GJ. Effect of pantoprazole on the course of reflux-associated laryngitis: a placebo-controlled double-blind crossover study. *Scand J Gastroenterol.* 2003;38(5):462–467.
27. El-Serag HB, Lee P, Buchner A, Inadomi JM, Gavin M, McCarthy DM. Lansoprazole treatment of patients with chronic idiopathic laryngitis: a placebo-controlled trial. *Am J Gastroenterol.* 2001;96(4):979–983.
28. Noordzij JP, Khidr A, Evans BA, et al. Evaluation of omeprazole in the treatment of reflux laryngitis: a prospective, placebo-controlled, randomized, double-blind study. *Laryngoscope.* 2001;111(12):2147–2151.

29. Steward DL. Pantoprazole for sleepiness associated with acid reflux and obstructive sleep disordered breathing. *Laryngoscope.* 2004;114(9):1525–1528.
30. Vaezi MF. Benefit of acid-suppressive therapy in chronic laryngitis: the devil is in the details. *Clin Gastroenterol Hepatol.* 2010;8(9):741–742.
31. Wo JM, Koopman J, Harrell SP, Parker K, Winstead W, Lentsch E. Double-blind, placebo-controlled trial with single-dose pantoprazole for laryngopharyngeal reflux. *Am J Gastroenterol.* 2006;101(9):1972–1978, quiz 2169.
32. Lam PK, Ng, ML, Cheung TK, et al. Rabeprazole is effective in treating laryngopharyngeal reflux in a randomized placebo-controlled trial. *Clin Gastroenterol Hepatol.* 2010;8(9):770–776.
33. Reichel O, Dressel H, Wiederänders K, Issing WJ. Double-blind, placebo-controlled trial with esomeprazole for symptoms and signs associated with laryngopharyngeal reflux. *Otolaryngol Head Neck Surg.* 2008;139(3):414–420.
34. Kahrilas PJ, Shaheen NJ, Vaezi MF, et al; American Gastroenterological Association. American Gastroenterological Association Medical position statement on the management of gastroesophageal reflux disease. *Gastroenterol.* 2008;135(4): 1381–1391.
35. Barry DW, Vaezi MF. Laryngopharyngeal reflux: more questions than answers. *Cleve Clin J Med.* 2010;77(5):327–334.
36. Gooi Z, Ishman SL, Bock JM, Blumin JH, Akst LM. Changing patterns in reflux care: 10-year comparison of ABEA members. *Ann Otol Rhinol Laryngol.* 2015; 124(12):940–946.
37. Lugaresi M, Aramini B, Daddi N, Baldi F, Mattioli S. Effectiveness of antireflux surgery for the cure of chronic cough associated with gastroesophageal reflux disease. *World J Surg.* 2015;39(1):208–215.
38. Faruqi S, Sedman P, Jackson W, Molyneux I, Morice AH. Fundoplication in chronic intractable cough. *Cough.* 2012;8(1):3.
39. Hoppo T, Komatsu Y, Jobe BA. Antireflux surgery in patients with chronic cough and abnormal proximal exposure as measured by hypopharyngeal multichannel intraluminal impedance. *JAMA Surg.* 2013;148(7):608–615.
40. Francis DO, Goutte M, Slaughter JC, et al. Traditional reflux parameters and not impedance monitoring predict outcome after fundoplication in extraesophageal reflux. *Laryngoscope.* 2011;121(9):1902–1909.
41. Tutuian R, Mainie I, Agrawal A, Adams D, Castell DO. Nonacid reflux in patients with chronic cough on acid-suppressive therapy. *Chest.* 2006;130(2):386–391.
42. Iqbal M, Batch AJ, Moorthy K, Cooper BT, Spychal RT. Outcome of surgical fundoplication for extra-oesophageal symptoms of reflux. *Surg Endosc.* 2009; 23(3):557–561.
43. Carroll TL, Nahikian K, Asban A, Wiener D. Nissen fundoplication for laryngopharyngeal reflux after patient selection using dual pH, full column impedance testing: a pilot study. *Ann Otol Rhinol Laryngol.* 2016;125(9):722–728.
44. Campagnolo AM, Priston J, Thoen RH, Medeiros T, Assunção AR. Laryngopharyngeal reflux: diagnosis, treatment, and latest research. *Int Arch Otorhinolaryngol.* 2014;18(2):184–191.
45. Hopwood D, Bateson MC, Milne G, Bouchier IA. Effects of bile acids and hydrogen ion on the fine structure of oesophageal epithelium. *Gut.* 1981;22(4):306–311.
46. Eto T, Tompkins RK. Further studies on the inhibition of pepsin by bile salts. *Ann Surg.* 1986;203(1):8–12.

47. Ali MS, Parikh S, Chater P, Pearson JP. Bile acids in laryngopharyngeal refluxate: will they enhance or attenuate the action of pepsin? *Laryngoscope.* 2013;123(2): 434–439.
48. Bardhan KD, Strugala V, Dettmar PW. Reflux revisited: advancing the role of pepsin. *Int J Otolaryngol.* 2012;2012:646901.
49. Francis DO, Rymer JA, Slaughter JC, et al. High economic burden of caring for patients with suspected extraesophageal reflux. *Am J Gastroenterol.* 2013;108(6): 905–911.
50. Belafsky PC. PRO: Empiric treatment with PPIs is not appropriate without testing. *Am J Gastroenterol.* 2006;101(1):6–8.
51. Carroll TL, Werner A, Nahikian K, Dezube A, Roth DF. Rethinking the laryngopharyngeal reflux treatment algorithm: evaluating an alternate empiric dosing regimen and considering up-front, pH-impedance, and manometry testing to minimize cost in treating suspect laryngopharyngeal reflux disease. *Laryngoscope.* 2017;127(suppl 6):S1–S13.

6

NEUROGENIC COUGH

John Paul Giliberto and Albert Merati

INTRODUCTION

Neurogenic cough is part of the wide differential diagnosis for patients presenting with chronic cough. Long considered a diagnosis of exclusion, neurogenic cough is often thought of when an initial evaluation for chronic cough does not identify a clear etiology.[1,2] The understanding of neurogenic cough as part of laryngeal hypersensitivity syndromes has progressed and, in the process, has undergone a number of nomenclature changes.[3,4] The following section of this chapter will review the literature on neurogenic cough and associated laryngeal hypersensitivity syndromes. Next, the chapter will review aspects of the patient history and exam, as well as other testing such as laryngeal visualization with stroboscopy and laryngeal electromyography (LEMG), both pertinent when considering a diagnosis of neurogenic cough. Finally, the evidence for treatment of neurogenic cough with both neuromodulating medications (neuromodulators) and speech therapy will be reviewed. The discussion of neuromodulators will include suggested dosing and titration schedules.

HISTORY OF NEUROGENIC COUGH AND LARYNGEAL HYPERSENSITIVITY SYNDROMES

Neurogenic cough denotes the symptom of chronic cough likely related to neuropathy or nerve dysfunction,[4] while laryngeal hypersensitivity syndrome (also known as cough hypersensitivity syndrome) encompasses a broader constellation of symptoms, including neurogenic cough, throat clearing, dysphonia, and dysphagia.[5] The suggestion that cough could be a manifestation of neuropathy or laryngeal hypersensitivity was first described as a part of ILS by Morrison et al (1999). The authors hypothesized that an acute traumatic event or a chronic noxious stimuli placed the larynx into a hyperfunctional, spasm-ready state.[3] Patients with ILS exhibit evidence of laryngeal hyperfunction (laryngospasm, dysphonia, globus, and cough) that can be reliably triggered by innocuous sensory stimuli (odors, food, voice use, exertion, or refluxate).[3] Although the most common proposed etiologic factor was gastroesophageal reflux, 17 out of 39 patients had a preceding viral illness.[3] Subsequent investigations have focused on the neurogenic manifestations of these laryngeal symptoms and evidence of vagal neuropathy. Linking the concepts of a neuropathy and antecedent viral illness, case series have described a postviral vagal neuropathy (PVVN) with symptoms that may include globus sensation, neurogenic chronic cough, vocal fold paresis, and dysphagia.[6–8] One of these studies, by Amin and Kaufman (2001), demonstrated laryngeal electromyographical evidence of neuropathy. Descriptions of PVVN have inclusion criteria of an antecedent viral illness, but other descriptions of ILS and laryngeal sensory neuropathies exhibit cases of vagal neuropathy without preceding viral illness.[3,6,7,9,10] In addition, Giliberto et al (2017) looked at predictors of response to treatment for neurogenic cough and noted no association between preceding viral illness and improved response to neuromodulator therapy, although the study population was small.[10]

Neurogenic cough associated with a PVVN limits the discussion of neurogenic coughs to those suspected to be viral in origin. In contrast, laryngeal sensory neuropathy (LSN) is a more general term used to describe chronic cough associated with evidence of vagal neuropathy.[1,9,11–13] Unfortunately, beyond subjective patient reports of laryngeal dysesthesias ("tickle"), objective evidence of vagal sensory neuropathy is limited or not readily available. Some authors have used capsaicin sensitivity testing, but changes in cough threshold are noted in the chronic cough population and not specific to patients with neurogenic cough.[14–16] Furthermore, limiting the discussion of cough as a sensory neuropathy fails to acknowledge that motor neuropathy was noted in 49% to 100% of patients in patient with both LSN and PVVN.[6,7,9] These studies have improved our current understanding of the interplay of neuropathy and chronic cough. With varied terminology in the literature, most authors favor the inclusive terminology of neurogenic cough for the symptoms of chronic cough thought to be related to vagal neuropathy and laryngeal hypersensitivity syndrome to encompass the syndrome of hyperfunctional laryngeal symptoms including cough, globus, throat clearing, and muscle tension associated with innocuous stimuli.[4,17–19]

PATHOPHYSIOLOGY

The act of coughing can be both a reflex requiring little conscious control and a voluntary act.[5] A discussion of neurogenic cough benefits from a brief review of the cough reflex and how it is thought to be affected in laryngeal hypersensitivity syndromes. The reflex is initiated by excitation of the sensory peripheral branches of the vagus nerve, originating from the mucosa of the larynx, pharynx, and esophagus.[20] Both noxious chemical stimuli (capsaicin or odors) and pressure can activate the afferent sensory nerve via chemosensitive nociceptors and mechanosensors, respectively.[5] In the healthy individual, these excitatory stimuli travel up afferent first-order neurons to the solitary nucleus in the brainstem.[4,5] Little is known about the exact physiology of sensory input integration and summation in the brainstem. Evidence in animal models demonstrates that frequent sensory nerve action potentials recruit N-methyl-D-aspartate (NMDA) receptors expressed on second-order nerves in the brainstem.[21] These second-order neurons are responsible for coordination of the respiratory motor response (ie, cough), but it is unclear how this may be augmented in the patient with neurogenic cough. Connections from the motor and sensory cortex to the solitary nucleus allow for volitional initiation and inhibition of coughing.[5]

It is hypothesized that in patients with neurogenic cough, this normal cough reflex is potentiated by three mechanisms. The first proposed mechanism involves lowering the threshold for activation of afferent sensory nerves. Antigen or viral inflammation in animal models leads to increase neuropeptide production and expression, thereby influencing the concentration of mechanoreceptors and nociceptors.[5] These changes can lower the threshold for activation of the sensory afferent nerve. In addition, these increased receptor expressions can lead to spontaneous activation, which underlies the second proposed mechanism. The sensation of phantom irritation of the throat, or the "bogus tickle," as stated by Bastian et al,[11] is often clinically noted in the setting of neurogenic cough. In the chronic pain literature, changes in afferent nerves, as noted above, can lead to spontaneous activation. However, similar spontaneous depolarizations have not been demonstrated in a cough model, nor have they been linked to laryngeal dysethesias.[5] A final mechanism of neurogenic cough involves an increase in the gain of the cough reflex at the brainstem level (or central sensitization).[4,5] Convergence of airway and esophageal sensory inputs can amplify incoming afferent sensations, augmenting the gain of the reflex. In addition, neuropeptides, such as substance P, have been shown to be upregulated following neural inflammation, and can produce durable excitatory effects on afferent nerves.[5] These proposed mechanisms exclude lesser-studied effects from muscular spasm and irritation from overstimulation, and do not include behavioral components such as habit, neurosis, and secondary gain.[22]

HISTORY AND PHYSICAL EXAM

As neurogenic cough has often been a diagnosis of exclusion, the focus of initial history and physical exam should be on symptoms and signs of other common etiologies, as detailed in previous chapters. It is important to keep in mind that many of the symptoms of a vagal neuropathy can be nonspecific and can cloud the clinical picture. For example, vagal nerve dysfunction can lead to dysphagia and esophageal dysmotility, resulting in heartburn and solid food dysphagia—symptoms more often associated with gastroesophageal reflux disease (GERD) than neurogenic cough. Reviewing the literature, prospective cohorts have identified elements of the patient history and physical exam that are associated with neurogenic cough. These elements include reliable cough triggers, antecedent viral illness, and evidence of laryngeal hyperfunction on physical exam. Although these elements may have limited sensitivity and specificity for neurogenic cough, they have evidence to support their association.

The description of hypersensitive larynx syndrome and ILS both cite benign triggers for neurogenic cough. These triggers include often innocuous stimuli such as odors, food, exercise, temperature changes, or speech.[3–5] As discussed in the pathophysiology section, a lower threshold for activation of afferent nerves of the larynx and pharynx could explain an overzealous reaction of the cough reflex to typically innocuous stimuli. Along with cough response to innocuous stimuli, the description of laryngeal hypersensitivity syndromes is associated with symptoms of globus, dysphonia, and laryngospasm. In Morrison's landmark paper describing ILS, 65% (25 out of 39) of patients had laryngospasm, 26% (10 out of 39) of patients experienced dysphonia, and 77% (30 out of 39) patients experienced cough or globus. Although present, these symptoms are not specific enough in the setting of chronic cough to suggest a neurogenic origin.

Patients with PVVN by definition have an antecedent vial illness, but other syndromes such as ILS cite antecedent viral illness in 17 out of 39 cases.[3,6–8] Many experts feel that acute onset of cough or other nonspecific symptoms of ILS following an upper respiratory illness can support a neurogenic origin of chronic cough. The larger PVVN description by Rees et al noted patients had persistent cough (52%), throat clearing (48%), dysphonia (41%), and other less-common complaints after upper respiratory illness.[7] Given that the presence of a preceding viral illness is required for inclusion in these studies, we cannot make conclusions about the frequency or association of neurogenic cough with antecedent upper respiratory illnesses. Other case series, not limited to PVVN, inconsistently report antecedent URI or do not have sufficient patient populations to note an association. A small retrospective study of patients suspected to have neurogenic cough looked at factors associated with response to neuromodulator therapy and did not demonstrate an association between viral illness and response to therapy; however, few patients in this study were reported to have an antecedent URI (four out of 25).[10]

Similar to the history, the absence of objective findings on physical exam of other etiologies of chronic cough is most consistent with neurogenic cough. Clinicians trained and familiar with palpation of the laryngeal muscles may find tension in the strap muscles, especially in the thyrohyoid space, suggesting laryngeal hyperfunction consistent with the description of, although not specific to, ILS.[3] Evidence of other upper cranial neuropathies may support the presence of a vagal neuropathy.[6] Evidence of motor neuropathy of the larynx and pharynx can be quite informative and will be discussed in the next section. Otherwise, there are few specific physical exam findings consistent with neurogenic cough.

In summary, there are myriad of clinical symptoms associated with neurogenic cough and laryngeal hypersensitivity syndrome. Complaints of globus, dysphonia, dysphagia, and throat clearing are not, in isolation, specific enough to indicate a neurogenic etiology of chronic coughing. However, there are historical elements and symptoms that, when taken in context of the whole clinical picture, may support the diagnosis of neurogenic cough. Expert reviews cite the presence of triggers (chemical, odors, mechanical, or temperature)[4] or antecedent viral illness[3,6,7] as the most specific elements of the history and physical supporting a diagnosis of neurogenic cough.

DIAGNOSTICS

Successful diagnosis of neurogenic cough requires laboratory and diagnostic testing to appropriately assess the wide differential of chronic cough. As with patient history and physical exam, negative findings for other etiologies of chronic cough can support a diagnosis of neurogenic cough. Chapter 9 will detail a comprehensive diagnostic approach to chronic cough, including the use of objective testing to evaluate pulmonary, sinonasal, and reflux-related causes in the context of the individual patient. Particularly germane to neurogenic cough is an evaluation of the larynx to rule out pathology and to evaluate for evidence of motor neuropathy. This can be accomplished with laryngoscopy with or without stroboscopy and LEMG. For providers not familiar with these procedures, the next section will give a brief overview of each procedure before moving on to how they can help with diagnosis and treatment.

LARYNGOSCOPY AND STROBOSCOPY

Visualization of the larynx can be performed indirectly with a mirror, or directly visualized through the use of a flexible fiberoptic laryngoscope or a rigid 70-degree endoscope. Although a trained and experienced examiner may be able to obtain a crisp and clear view of the larynx with a mirror through indirect laryngoscopy, the ability to record and obtain reliable images with superior image resolution has led many otolaryngologists to favor either flexible fiberoptic, distal chip digital, or rigid transoral laryngoscopy.[23] Flexible laryngoscopy is the more common modality and is well tolerated by patients in the setting of an office visit, with or without topical anesthesia to the nose.[23,24] Once the scope traverses the nose, it provides a view of the oropharynx, hypopharynx, and larynx. The scope delivers light via fiberoptic fibers, and the images are returned by additional fibers or a distal CCD chip via wire. These images can be recorded on video capture systems, allowing for slow-motion review and storage for later comparison. Rigid Hopkins rod laryngoscopes (70- or 90-degree) are introduced through the mouth over the tongue and visualize the larynx with a camera attached as an image-capture device. Laryngoscopy (either flexible or rigid) can be performed using a special lighting protocol called stroboscopy. In this case, light from the scope is pulsed at a frequency just slightly different than the patient's fundamental frequency. This pulsed light provides a sequence of images that can give the illusion (or simulation) of a slow-motion view of the glottic vibratory cycle as long as the patient can maintain a consistent and periodic vibration.[23] The addition of this simulated slow motion allows for assessment of vibration of the vocal folds and their closure pattern.The improved optics allow for assessment of mucosal lesions and subtle differences in motion. Although rigid endoscopes provide excellent video quality of the vibrating vocal folds during stroboscopic light imaging, they cannot assess vocal fold motion during connected speech.[23,24]

Findings on laryngoscopy and stroboscopy are subjective; however, certain diagnoses have different interrater reliabilities. While many examiners can agree on the side of vocal fold immobility and paralysis, evidence of subtle paresis is more difficult to ascertain as to which is the affected side.[25,26] Signs on stroboscopy of vocal fold paresis include asymmetry in mucosal wave, motion asymmetry, laryngeal axis rotation, compensatory supraglottic hyperfunction, and glottic insufficiency.[25,27] Although motion or vibratory abnormalities are not reliable predictors of side of injury, both Simpson et al (2011) and Woo et al (2016) showed that physicians correctly diagnosed the presence of asymmetry stroboscopy 83% and 88% of the time, respectively.[25,26] Thus, when performed by an experienced provider, laryngoscopy with stroboscopy has a good association with the presence of neuropathy, but poor reliability as to which side is weak.

Many cough patients benefit from the involvement by an otolaryngologist or laryngologist for evaluation of the larynx and hypopharynx. A flexible exam with stroboscopy by an experienced interpreter will likely provide a thorough assessment of vocal fold motion asymmetries consistent with motor neuropathy. The presence of motor neuropathy on stroboscopy or, as will be discussed in the next section, on LEMG can support the presence of a vagal neuropathy. This may be helpful in narrowing the differential diagnosis and supporting a diagnosis of neurogenic cough.

LARYNGEAL ELECTROMYOGRAPHY

LEMG is a procedural evaluation technique of muscle fiber action potentials and motor unit action potentials in the laryngeal muscles.[28] Typically, it is performed under local anesthesia in the office by a laryngologist, neurologist, or physical medicine and rehabilitation electromyographer, or two of these providers together. After local anesthesia, a needle electrode is advanced into the laryngeal muscles and morphology of the action potentials are qualitatively or quantitatively evaluated for signs of acute or chronic injury,[28,29] the details of which are beyond the scope of this chapter. Some groups perform qualitative analysis to help quantify degree of injury and standardize diagnosis. However, the practice of LEMG remains varied as does the ability of providers to incorporate it into a regular outpatient clinic, as some providers may need to schedule an LEMG weeks or months following an initial evaluation. Although the qualitative assessment of motor neuropathy on LEMG has a subjective component, the data from LEMG are felt to be more objective than the finding of laryngoscopy with stroboscopy. LEMG is often used as the gold standard to compare laryngoscopy findings when evaluating sensitivity and specificity of clinician ratings for subtle paresis.[25,26]

Motor Neuropathy and Choosing the Diagnostic Modality

Stroboscopy and LEMG can be used to assess a patient with neurogenic cough for associated motor neuropathy that may suggest a neurologic change has occured. Studies of neurogenic cough often include videostroboscopy results,[10,13,30] but others include evidence from both LEMG and stroboscopic modalities.[6,9] In the two retrospective case series and one prospective consecutive cohort that looked at response to medical treatment, all studies demonstrated improved response to treatment in patients with motor neuropathy (Table 6–1). In considering the decision for LEMG and stroboscopy, the latter is far more readily available than LEMG in the evaluation of neurogenic cough. In addition, beyond looking for the presence of motor neuropathy, flexible laryngoscopy and stroboscopy can be helpful in focusing the differential and ruling out laryngeal pathology as the source of the chronic cough. Thus, given its availability, tolerability, and benefit to the cough differential, stroboscopy is often performed in the evaluation of chronic cough.

Table 6–1. Motor Neuropathy and Neuromodulator Response. Review of the studies that evaluated patients for evidence of motor neuropathy and response to neuromodulator therapy

		Improvement with Neuromodulator Therapy? n/total (%)	
First Author (Year)	Evidence of Motor Neuropathy	Evidence of Motor Neuropathy	No Evidence of Motor Neuropathy
Norris (2010)[13]	Stroboscopy	9/9 (100%)*	1/3 (33%)*
Giliberto (2017)[10]	Stroboscopy	16/20 (80%)	1/5 (20%)
Lee (2005)[9]	Stroboscopy and LEMG	15/18 (83%)	3/8 (38%)

LEMG = Laryngeal electromyography.

*Proportion difference reported without statistical evaluation.

TREATMENT

Once the diagnosis of neurogenic cough is clinically suspected, randomized controlled trials have shown that the use of neuromodulating medications can improve cough severity[8,31,32] and cough-related quality of life.[8,31,32] Neuromodulators with level 1 evidence include gabapentin, amitriptyline, and pregabalin.[8,31,32] Other agents, including tramadol and baclofen, have been used with success.[33,34] In addition, cough retraining therapy by a trained speech-language pathologist may play a role in treatment and maintaining effective treatment, as discussed in Chapter 8.[31] A number of questions remain around the treatment of chronic cough with neuromodulators, including: what is the most effective agent, what are the optimal dose/titration regimens (Table 6–2), what are adequate lengths for therapy, and what are the long-term outcomes. Following a review of the literature on specific agents, this chapter will answer these questions.

Motor Neuropathy and Choosing the Diagnostic Modality

Amitriptyline

Amitriptyline is a tricyclic antidepressant (TCA) that mainly inhibits both serotonin and norepinephrine reuptake but may weakly interact with several other receptors including opioid, adenosine, α_2-adrenergic, NMDA, nicotinic, cholinergic, and histaminergic receptors.[35] With respect to TCAs, amitriptyline also has prominent anticholinergic effects, which should be considered in elderly patients. In the prospective studies listed in Table 6–2,

Table 6–2. Reported Neuromodulator Dosing Regimens

First Author (Year)	Agent	Medication Regimen	Titration?
Bastian (2006)[11]	Amitriptyline	10 mg daily for 3 wks.	No
Jeyakumar (2006)[8]	Amitriptyline	10 mg daily for 10 d.	No
Norris (2010)[13]	Amitriptyline	Start at 25 mg qHS, increased to maximum of 100 mg qHS.†	Yes*
Ryan (2016)[41]	Amitriptyline	Start at 10 mg qHS, increase daily dose by 10 mg each wk, to maximum dose of 100 mg qHS.	Yes*
Dicpinigaitis (1998)[34]	Baclofen	10 mg TID for 14 d.	No
Lee (2005)[5]	Gabapentin	Start at 100 mg daily, increase over 4 wks to 900 mg, divided TID. If effective maintain dose for 3 m.	Yes*
Mintz (2006)[43]	Gabapentin	Start at 100 mg BID, increased to max daily dose of 1600 mg.†	Yes*
Ryan (2012)[32]	Gabapentin	Start 300 mg daily, increase daily dose by 300 mg each d to max daily dose of 1800 mg (divided TID). Maintain dose for 10 wks, then taper over 7 d.	Yes*
Halum (2009)[12]	Pregabalin	Start at 75 mg BID, increase over 4 wks to 150 mg BID‡, maintain for at least 1 m.	Yes*
Vertigan (2016)[31]	Pregabalin	Start at 75 mg increased to 300 mg daily dose, divided TID. Maintain dose for 11 wks.	Yes*
Dion (2017)[33]	Tramadol	50 mg TID PRN for 2 wks.	No

d = day, wk = week, m = month, BID = twice daily, TID = three times daily, qHS = daily at night, PRN = take as needed for cough symptoms.

*Dose was titrated to cough symptom resolution or adverse effect that were not tolerable.

†Titration schedule and treatment length not reported.

‡One patient required pregabalin 150 mg TID to obtain complete symptom relief.

amitriptyline has been shown to improve cough symptoms in 75% to 83% of patients. A randomized placebo-controlled trial conducted by Jeyakumar et al (2006) demonstrated significant improvement in cough severity and cough-related quality of life with a 10-day course.[8]

Many physicians favor amitriptyline because it demonstrates predictable efficacy and once-daily dosing regimens (see Table 6–3 for a suggested titration, and Table 6–2 for other published dosing regimens). However,

Table 6–3. Suggested Titration Schedule for Amitriptyline

	Week	Evening
Escalation* with 10 mg tablets (Disp #70)	1	10 mg
	2	2 × 10 mg
	3	3 × 10 mg
	4	4 × 10 mg
Follow-up		
Escalation* with 25 mg tablets (Disp #91)	5	2 × 25 mg
	6	3 × 25 mg
	7	4 × 25 mg
	8	4 × 25 mg

Table is for escalation of titration. De-escalation can be much quicker, decreasing 1 capsule per day.

mg = milligrams, Disp = dispense # capsules for the month titration.

*Dose titrated to cough symptom resolution or adverse effect.

concerns regarding anticholinergic effects of amitriptyline in patients over 65 years old may put these patients at increased risk of adverse effects. Based on the BEERS criteria for potentially harmful medications in older adults, strongly anticholinergic TCAs, such as amitriptyline, have led the American Geriatric Society to state that the use of these medications in patients over age 65 is potentially harmful.[36] With this in mind, many experts have turned to nortriptyline as a substitute and, anecdotally, it has similar efficacy with less anticholinergic effects. However, efficacy of nortriptyline has not been established in either prospective or retrospective studies for chronic neurogenic cough.

Gabapentin and Pregablin

Both gabapentin and pregabalin are GABA analogs, and their mechanism of action is to inhibit voltage-gated calcium-channel neurotransmitter release.[4] Both agents have level 1 evidence supporting their use in neurogenic cough, and many consider both as first-line agents to treat neurogenic cough.[4,9] With its long history of treatment of neuropathy, initial studies on the effectiveness of GABA analogs focused on gabapentin. In a prospective case series of 28 consecutive patients, Lee and Woo (2005) evaluated the effect of gabapentin on patients with laryngeal sensory neuropathy, specifically on symptoms of cough, dysphagia, globus, and laryngospasm. All patients were evaluated with stroboscopy and LEMG for evidence of motor neuropathy, which was noted in 20 out of 28 patients (71%).[9] Dichotomous yes/no improvement in cough symptoms was noted in 69% of all patients and in 80% of patients with evidence of motor neuropathy (see Table 6–1). Ryan et al (2012) performed a randomized double-blind placebo-controlled study that evaluated gabapentin's effect on cough severity and cough-related quality of life. Not only was there a noted improvement in cough severity as measured by a visual analog scale and a cough monitor, but there was also a noted clinical and statistical improvement in cough severity in the gabapentin treatment arm.[32] Ultimately, however, 4 weeks after discontinuation of the course of gabapentin, there failed to be a durable improvement in cough-related quality of life and severity between the two groups.[32] Table 6–4 delineates a suggested gabapentin titration, but there are many other dosing regimens, as seen in Table 6–2.

Similar to gabapentin, pregabalin has prospective case series data and a randomized control trial to support its efficacy. In a randomized control trial by Vertigan et al (2016), the experimental arm of the study included four sessions of speech therapy with a titration of pregabalin, and the control was a placebo and four sessions of speech therapy. Clinically and statistically significant improvement in cough severity and related quality of life was noted at completion of treatment in the therapy plus pregabalin group, compared to therapy alone with placebo. At follow-up 18 weeks later there was no longer a difference between the experimental and control groups in cough-related quality of life and cough severity, but both the treatment and placebo had improved compared to baseline measures.[31] The

Table 6–4. Suggested Titration Schedule for Gabapentin

	Week	Morning	Midday	Evening
Escalation* with 100 mg Capsules (Disp #126)	1	100 mg	100 mg	100 mg
	2	100 mg	100 mg	2 × 100 mg
	3	100 mg	2 × 100 mg	2 × 100 mg
	4	2 × 100 mg	2 × 100 mg	2 × 100 mg
Follow-up				
Escalation* with 300 mg Capsules (Disp #126)	5	300 mg	300 mg	300 mg
	6	300 mg	300 mg	2 × 300 mg
	7	300 mg	2 × 300 mg	2 × 300 mg
	8	2 × 300 mg	2 × 300 mg	2 × 300 mg

Table is for escalation of titration. De-escalation can be much quicker, decreasing 1 capsule per day.
mg = milligrams, Disp = dispense # capsules for the month titration.
*Dose titrated to cough symptom resolution or adverse effect.

Table 6–5. Suggested Titration Schedule for Pregabalin

	Day	Morning	Midday	Evening
	1–2	75 mg		
Escalation*	3–4	75 mg		75 mg
	5–6	75 mg	75 mg	75 mg
	7–84	75 mg	75 mg	150 mg
	85–86	75 mg	75 mg	75 mg
De-escalation	87–88	75 mg		75 mg
	89–90	75 mg		

Modified from data presented by Vertigan et al (2016).[31]

mg = milligrams.

*Dose titrated to cough symptom resolution or adverse effects that were not tolerable.

pregabalin titration schedule from this study is detailed in Table 6–5, but other reported dosing schedules are available in Table 6–2.

Other Agents

Baclofen and tramadol are other neuromodulators that have been used successfully in case series to treat neurogenic cough, and are considered alternatives if first-line agents are not effective.[4] Baclofen has been shown to blunt the cough reflex and cough stimulation with a capsaicin challenge;[37] however, data for use in neurogenic cough is limited to a two-person crossover case report. Both patients had decreased cough severity with 2 weeks of baclofen. Tramadol, a weak opioid receptor agonist, has demonstrated benefit in both cough-related quality of life scores and cough severity in a prospective cohort in a study performed by Dion et al in 2017. Although this confirmed what many experts anecdotally noted regarding benefit, the follow-up was limited, leaving questions of long-term benefit.[33] In addition, being a weak opioid agonist, there is concern regarding chemical dependence, which has been demonstrated in doses as low as 50 mg per day.[38] Being the only schedule IV drug on this neuromodulator list, there are also logistical issues and state regulations to be aware of when writing tramadol prescriptions, including requirements to consult state narcotic prescriptions databases, limits on electronic or called-in prescriptions, and refill limits. Many of these requirements vary by state and are changing as states try to address the opioid epidemic; reviewing state requirements is prudent before incorporating tramadol into routine clinical use. Dosing regimens can be found in Table 6–2.

INITIAL AGENT SELECTION

With limited and varied study designs and lack of side-by-side comparisons, a systemic review by Cohen and Misono (2013) failed to identify a superior agent, length of therapy, or follow-up course.[2] Preferences for agents, therefore, exist mostly based on other factors besides efficacy. Many authors consider gabapentin, amitriptyline, and pregabalin as first-line agents.[4,12,13,18] Between these three agents, amitriptyline has the benefit of once-daily dosing, but with its anticholinergic activity it should be used cautiously in adults older than 65. Many have substituted nortriptyline in this patient population, but it lacks the data to support its efficacy. Amitriptyline can also interact with selective serotonin reuptake inhibitors or other serotonergic medications to cause serotonin syndrome.[39] For these reasons, other providers favor gabapentin or pregabalin as their first-line agent despite the three times daily dosing. With the limited data on tramadol and baclofen, these are considered only after failing one, two or three of the first-line agents.

TITRATION, ADVERSE EFFECTS AND LONG-TERM OUTCOMES

All of the first-line medications have large therapeutic ranges, and many published regimens include a titration, although there are no accepted rates of titration or maximum doses (see Table 6–2). Adverse effects were common and are delineated agent by agent in Table 6–6. Serious medication complications were not observed, and any adverse effects resolved with cessation of the neuromodulator.[18] With the frequency of adverse effects ranging from 17% to 75% (see Table 6–6), medication titration allows for identification of a dosage with cough symptoms, minimizing chances for adverse effects. Many authors employ a titration in the prescribed regimen as delineated in Table 6–2. There is no consensus on optimal titration rate, or length or course of therapy.[4] It has been the practice of the author of this chapter to continue patients on treatment for 3 to 6 months before a trial wean and discontinuation of medications, which is consistent with use of neuromodulators in the chronic pain literature.[40]

With initial benefit of neuromodulators well established, authors have turned their attention to long-term outcomes for therapy. Some patients may need treatment indefinitely, while others may have durable benefits following a 3- to 6-month course of optimal dosing.[4,41] In Ryan et al (2012), cough severity and cough-related quality of life improved initially; however, 1 month after gabapentin was discontinued, this improvement was no longer present. In the only study of long-term follow-up, Ryan et al (2016) surveyed 36 patients with neurogenic cough treated with amitriptyline about their long-term results and continued medication usage.[41]

Table 6–6. Reported Neuromodulator Adverse Effects

First Author (Year)	Agent	Adverse Effects	Therapy Discontinued*
Bastian (2006)[11]	Amitriptyline	NR	NR
Jeyakumar (2006)[8]	Amitriptyline	NR	NR
Norris (2010)[13]	Amitriptyline	Dry mouth (30%)	1/12 (8.3%)
Ryan (2016)[41]	Amitriptyline	Sedation (11%), increased appetite (2.8%), pain in lymph nodes (2.8%)	1/36 (2.8%)
Dicpinigaitis (1998)[34]	Baclofen	NR	NR
Lee (2005)[5]	Gabapentin	Dizziness or somnolence (17.8%)	NR
Mintz (2006)[43]	Gabapentin	Fatigue (17%)	0/6
Ryan (2012)[32]	Gabapentin	Total (31%) including blurred vision, disorientation, confusion, dizziness, dry mouth, fatigue, headache, memory loss, and nausea; versus placebo (10%)	1/26 (4%) in gabapentin and 1/24 (4%) placebo group
Halum (2009)[12]	Pregabalin	Somnolence/mental fog (33.3%), worsening of preexisting leg pain (8.3%)	2/12 (17%)
Vertigan (2016)[31]	Pregabalin	Total (75%) including blurred vision, cognitive changes, dizziness, dry mouth, fatigue, headache, gastrointestinal, weight gain, skin, fluid buildup; versus placebo (75%)	1/20 (5%) fall
Dion (2017)[33]	Tramadol	Somnolence (25%)	0/16 (0%)

*Neuromodulatory therapy was discontinued because patients experienced side effects. Does not include patients who continue to get benefits from lower dose.

At 2 to 3 years after completion of treatment, 20 out of 38 (53%) maintained the ≥50% cough reduction, but of those 20 patients, 11 were still taking amitriptyline at the time of the follow-up survey.[41]

BEHAVIORAL COUGH REDUCTION

The role of the SLP and cough suppression/retraining techniques will be further discussed in Chapter 8; however, a brief discussion of speech therapy is germane to a review of neurogenic cough. A randomized, single-blinded, placebo-controlled trial looking at speech therapy versus healthy lifestyle education showed an 88% improvement in cough severity in the experimental group compared to 13% in the control group.[42] Furthermore, four sessions of speech therapy were incorporated into both arms of the pregabalin randomized, double-blinded, placebo-controlled trial discussed above. Interestingly, benefit in cough severity and cough-related quality of life were preserved beyond cessation of both treatment arms when neuromodulators were combined with speech therapy, while the use of neuromodulators alone demonstrated lack of durable improvement.[31,32] Both of these randomized controlled studies were performed with different agents and were not set up to answer the question of speech therapy's effectiveness for neurogenic cough directly. The authors suggest that speech therapy may be responsible for the durable improvement in outcomes; however, further evidence looking specifically at the role of speech therapy with and without neuromodulator treatment will be needed to support this hypothesis.[31]

THINKING OUTSIDE OF THE BOX

Over the past two to three decades, our understanding of cough, outside of a respiratory infection, has progressed from a behavioral tick to a part of a syndrome such as ILS, laryngeal hypersensitivity syndrome, or PVVN. The understanding of laryngeal hypersensitivity syndrome and analogies to chronic pain have improved our understanding of neuropathic changes that can augment the cough reflex at the brainstem. In addition, the recognition that cough may be the result of a vagal neuropathy has lent itself to effective treatment with neuromodulators. Despite this understanding and effective treatment, for the most part neurogenic cough remains a diagnosis of exclusion and lacks criteria for a positive diagnosis based on present symptoms. This lack of diagnostic criteria not only makes a consensus of what constitutes neurogenic cough difficult for research purposes but also can lead to delays in diagnosis that can be months, years, and even decades long. As with any diagnosis of exclusion, the need for more specific tests to rule in or out the other common etiologies for chronic cough are needed. Fortunately, the ability to rule in or out allergies, reflux, and glottic insufficiency is becoming more commonplace. For example, the ability to rule reflux in or out has improved thanks to impedance testing that can demonstrate liquid reflux events of any pH from the lower esophagus up to and beyond the upper esophageal sphincter. Because true reflux due to post-viral vagal neuropathic effects on the upper GI tract can coexist in patients with vocal fold motion abnormalities in the setting of PVVN, it may be prudent to consider esophageal-hypopharyngeal impedance with dual pH testing in patients with other reflux related symptoms to determine if risk for esophageal damage is present, even in the setting of patients who respond to neuromodulator therapy.

Many experts, including the authors of this chapter, believe factors such as antecedent respiratory illness, unilateral globus or pain, acute onset, laryngeal dysesthesias, and evidence of laryngeal motor neuropathy are consistent with a clinical picture of neurogenic cough. Furthermore, the presence of these factors without strong evidence for alternative cough etiologies can prompt an initial trial of treatment for neurogenic cough before an extensive workup for other common etiologies of chronic cough. That being said, only evidence of motor neuropathy has been associated with response to neuromodulator therapy. Prospective studies looking at the association of these factors with cough are necessary to substantiate these conjectures and hopefully assemble criteria to dismiss the conjecture that neurogenic cough is a diagnosis of exclusion.

Until such research is available, when a careful systematic history-taking and physical and diagnostic workup do not obviously point to asthma, allergies, or reflux, consideration of neurogenic cough and a trial of one or two neuromodulators is warranted.

TAKE-HOME POINTS

- Laryngeal hypersensitivity syndromes including ILS, LSN, and PVVN have chronic neurogenic cough as a symptom.
- Neurogenic cough is classically considered a diagnosis of exclusion.
- Neurogenic cough may present in isolation, but can be associated with antecedent respiratory illness, globus, dysphagia, laryngospasm, laryngeal dysesthesias, and dysphonia.
- Stroboscopy and laryngeal electromyography can provide evidence of motor neuropathy, consistent with a possible neurogenic etiology of chronic cough.
- Neurogenic cough responds well to neuromodulators, but adverse effects are common.
- There is insufficient data to determine a superior initial choice of neuromodulating medication; first-line agents include gabapentin, amitriptyline, and pregabalin.

- Dosage and schedules for the various neuromodulator vary, and titration over days or weeks may provide cough relief while minimize adverse effects.
- Length of therapy and long-term efficacy of neuromodulators for neurogenic cough are not well known.
- There is likely a benefit of speech therapy, specifically working on respiratory retraining and cough suppression techniques, in conjunction with neuromodulator therapy in the treatment of neurogenic cough.

REFERENCES

1. Greene SM, Simpson CB. Evidence for sensory neuropathy and pharmacologic management. *Otolaryngol Clin North Am.* 2010;43(1):67–72, viii.
2. Cohen SM, Misono S. Use of specific neuromodulators in the treatment of chronic, idiopathic cough: a systematic review. *Otolaryngol Head Neck Surg.* 2013;148(3):374–382.
3. Morrison M, Rammage L, Emami AJ. The irritable larynx syndrome. *J Voice.* 1999;13(3):447–455.
4. Altman KW, Noordzij JP, Rosen CA, Cohen S, Sulica L. Neurogenic cough. *Laryngoscope.* 2015;125(7):1675–1681.
5. Chung KF, McGarvey L, Mazzone SB. Chronic cough as a neuropathic disorder. *Lancet Respir Med.*, 2013;1(5):414–422.
6. Amin MR, Koufman JA. Vagal neuropathy after upper respiratory infection: a viral etiology? *Am J Otolaryngol.*2001;22(4):251–256.
7. Rees CJ, Henderson AH, Belafsky PC. Postviral vagal neuropathy. *Ann Otol Rhinol Laryngol.* 2009;118(4):247–252.
8. Jeyakumar A, Brickman TM, Haben M. Effectiveness of amitriptyline versus cough suppressants in the treatment of chronic cough resulting from postviral vagal neuropathy. *Laryngoscope.* 2006;116(12):2108–2112.
9. Lee B, Woo P. Chronic cough as a sign of laryngeal sensory neuropathy: diagnosis and treatment. *Ann Otol Rhinol Laryngol.* 2005;114(4):253–257.
10. Giliberto JP, Dibildox D, Merati A. Unilateral laryngoscopic findings associated with response to gabapentin in patients with chronic cough. *JAMA Otolaryngol Head Neck Surg.* 2017;143(11):1081–1085.
11. Bastian RW, Vaidya AM, Delsupehe KG. Sensory neuropathic cough: a common and treatable cause of chronic cough. *Otolaryngol Head Neck Surg.* 2006;135(1):17–21.
12. Halum SL, Sycamore DL, McRae BR. A new treatment option for laryngeal sensory neuropathy. *Laryngoscope.* 2009;119(9):1844–1847.
13. Norris BK, Schweinfurth JM. Management of recurrent laryngeal sensory neuropathic symptoms. *Ann Otol Rhinol Laryngol.* 2010;119(3):188–191.
14. Sumner H, Woodcock A, Kolsum U, et al. Predictors of objective cough frequency in chronic obstructive pulmonary disease. *Am J Respir Crit Care Med.* 2013;187(9):943–949.

15. Kanezaki M, Ebihara S, Gui P, Ebihara T, Kohzuki M. Effect of cigarette smoking on cough reflex induced by TRPV1 and TRPA1 stimulations. *Respir Med.* 2012;106(3):406–412.
16. Doherty MJ, Mister R, Pearson MG, Calverley PM. Capsaicin responsiveness and cough in asthma and chronic obstructive pulmonary disease. *Thorax.* 2000;55(8):643–649.
17. Bock JM, Koszewski IJ, Blumin JH, et al. Surface-evoked laryngeal sensory action potential evaluation in neurogenic chronic cough. *J Voice.* 2014;28(5):624–630.
18. Giliberto JP, Cohen SM, Misono S. Are neuromodulating medications effective for the treatment of chronic neurogenic cough? [published online ahead of print Nov 15, 2016]. *Laryngoscope.*
19. Lim K. Neurogenic cough. *J Allergy Clin Immunol.* 2014;133(6):1779–e1773.
20. Lang IM, Medda BK, Babaei A, Shaker R. Role of peripheral reflexes in the initiation of the esophageal phase of swallowing. *Am J Physiol Gastrointest Liver Physiol.* 2014;306(8):G728–G737.
21. Canning BJ, Mori N. Encoding of the cough reflex in anesthetized guinea pigs. *Am J Physiol Regul Integr Comp Physiol.* 2011;300(2):R369–R377.
22. Altman JI, Genden EM, Moche J. Fiberoptic endoscopic-assisted diverticulotomy: a novel technique for the management of Zenker's diverticulum. *Ann Otol Rhinol Laryngol.* 2005;114(5):347–351.
23. Sulica L. Laryngoscopy, stroboscopy and other tools for the evaluation of voice disorders. *Otolaryngol Clin North Am.* 2013;46(1):21–30.
24. Merati AL, Rieder AA. Normal endoscopic anatomy of the pharynxand larynx. *Am J Med.* 2003;115(3):10–14.
25. Simpson CB, May LS, Green JK, Eller RL, Jackson CE. Vibratory asymmetry in mobile vocal folds: is it predictive of vocal fold paresis? *Ann Otol Rhinol Laryngol.* 2011;120(4):239–242.
26. Woo P, Isseroff TF, Parasher A, Richards A, Sivak M. Laryngeal electromyographic findings in patients with vocal fold motion asymmetry. *Laryngoscope.* 2016;126(8):E273–277.
27. Sulica L, Blitzer A. Vocal fold paresis: evidence and controversies. *Curr Opin Otolaryngol Head Neck Surg.* 2007;15(3):159–162.
28. Blitzer A, Crumley RL, Dailey SH, et al. Recommendations of the Neurolaryngology Study Group on laryngeal electromyography. *Otolaryngol Head Neck Surg.* 2009;140(6):782–793.
29. Statham MM, Rosen CA, Nandedkar SD, Munin MC. Quantitative laryngeal electromyography: turns and amplitude analysis. *Laryngoscope.* 2010;120(10):2036–2041.
30. Belafsky PC, Rees CJ, Allen J, Leonard RJ. Pharyngeal dilation in cricopharyngeus muscle dysfunction and Zenker diverticulum. *Laryngoscope.* 2010;120(5):889–894.
31. Vertigan AE, Kapela SL, Ryan NM, Birring SS, McElduff P, Gibson PG. Pregabalin and speech pathology combination therapy for refractory chronic cough: a randomized controlled trial. *Chest.* 2016;149(3):639–648.
32. Ryan NM, Birring SS, Gibson PG. Gabapentin for refractory chronic cough: a randomised, double-blind, placebo-controlled trial. *Lancet.* 2012;380(9853):1583–1589.
33. Dion GR, Teng SE, Achlatis E, Fang Y, Amin MR. Treatment of neurogenic cough with tramadol: a pilot study. *Otolaryngol Head Neck Surg.* 2017;157(1):77–79.

34. Dicpinigaitis PV, Rauf K. Treatment of chronic, refractory cough with baclofen. *Respiration.* 1998;65(1):86–88.
35. Fridrich P, Colvin HP, Zizza A, et al. Phase 1A safety assessment of intravenous amitriptyline. *J Pain.* 2007;8(7):549–555.
36. American Geriatrics Society Beers Criteria Update Expert Panel. American Geriatrics Society updated Beers Criteria for potentially inappropriate medication use in older adults. *J Am Geriatr Soc.* 2012;60(4):616–631.
37. Dicpinigaitis PV, Dobkin JB, Rauf K, Aldrich TK. Inhibition of capsaicin-induced cough by the gamma-aminobutyric acid agonist baclofen. *J Clin Pharmacol.* 1998;38(4):364–367.
38. Tjaderborn M, Jonsson AK, Ahlner J, Hagg S. Tramadol dependence: a survey of spontaneously reported cases in Sweden. *Pharmacoepidemiol Drug Saf.* 2009; 18(12):1192–1198.
39. Ferguson JM. SSRI antidepressant medications: adverse effects and tolerability. *Prim Care Companion J Clin Psychiatry.* 2001;3(1):22–27.
40. Dworkin RH, O'Connor AB, Audette J, et al. Recommendations for the pharmacological management of neuropathic pain: an overview and literature update. *Mayo Clin Proc.* 2010;85(suppl 3), S3–S14.
41. Ryan MA, Cohen SM. Long-term follow-up of amitriptyline treatment for idiopathic cough. *Laryngoscope.* 2016;126(12):2758-2763.
42. Vertigan AE, Theodoros DG, Gibson PG, Winkworth AL. Efficacy of speech pathology management for chronic cough: a randomised placebo controlled trial of treatment efficacy. *Thorax.* 2006;61(12):1065–1069.
43. Mintz S., & Lee, J. K. (2005). Gabapentin in the treatment of intractable idiopathic chronic cough: Case reports. *Am J Med,* 119(5), e13–e15.

7

DYSPHAGIA IN CHRONIC COUGH

Mark A. Fritz, Debra M. Suiter, and Gregory N. Postma

INTRODUCTION

Patients who present with chronic cough often have complaints of difficulty swallowing. The cough may be related to their swallowing dysfunction from an underlying etiology found in the laryngopharynx or esophagus and may be their only symptom. Aspiration or penetration of liquids or food into the larynx causes a profound cough reflex in the normal individual as a protective mechanism to prevent particles from entering the sterile respiratory system. When aspiration becomes pathologic, causing symptomatic cough or, more significantly, aspiration pneumonia, the significance of treating the patient goes from a quality-of-life issue to a lifesaving one.

There are many reasons why a patient may present with both dysphagia and cough symptoms. The most common reason a patient feels both cough and difficulty swallowing is reflux disease, and this is covered in depth in Chapter 4. Postviral vagal neuropathy can occur following a viral infection, such as an upper respiratory infection, and can present with a number of aerodigestive symptoms including cough; this is discussed in Chapter 5.[1,2] Both the motor and the sensory branches of the vagus nerve can be affected, and patients often report complaints of globus sensation, throat irritation, dysphonia, throat clearing, and throat tightness.[3] Additionally, patients may present with a cough and complaints of dysphagia following intubation or after a cerebrovascular accident, both with much higher potential for morbidity than the aforementioned. A screening examination is performed, most commonly by a speech-language pathologist, to determine if a patient's swallowing and cough reflexes are appropriately intact to prevent a devastating aspiration event before oral feeding is resumed.

Accurate assessment of individuals with aspiration due to oropharyngeal dysphagia is critically important. Unrecognized dysphagia can lead to serious health consequences for patients, including dehydration, malnutrition, aspiration pneumonia, and even death. When a patient presents with complaints of dysphagia in the setting of a chronic cough, it is important to determine if those complaints are consistent with oropharyngeal or esophageal dysphagia and not presumed to be due to reflux disease. In this chapter, we will review assessment of oropharyngeal and esophageal swallowing in patients with chronic cough.

DYSPHAGIA SCREENING

Patients with swallowing problems and chronic cough will often be treated at minimum by an otolaryngologist and a speech-language pathologist (SLP). Patients in the hospital with new-onset dysphagia will typically have a screening first to evaluate for swallow impairment (see the following bulleted list). Conversely, in the outpatient setting, patients find their way to either an SLP or an otolaryngologist, depending on referral patterns. The team approach to these complicated and medically ill patients is important for both diagnosis and intervention. Additional specialties that are often involved with the treatment of dysphagia with concomitant chronic cough include pulmonologists, gastroenterologists, and neurologists.

When a patient presents with chronic cough, dysphagia symptoms should be explored and pursued further if necessary. High-yield questions include:

- Do you have any problem swallowing solid foods?
- Do you experience choking or aspirating on liquids?
- Are you losing weight?
- Do you have to avoid any specific foods?
- Have you ever received radiation treatment to the head and/or neck?
- Do you have any history of respiratory infections, including pneumonia?
- Do you have any history of head and neck surgery?
- Do you ever regurgitate your food?

A positive response to any of these questions can suggest dysphagia that warrants workup to determine any contribution of dysphagia to the patient's chronic cough. The otolaryngologist should always perform flexible laryngoscopy for the patient with chronic cough or dysphagia, as it will show anatomic changes that may explain the issues, such as a laryngeal mass, large glottic gap with or without vocal fold paralysis, or a large amount of pooling in the pyriform sinuses. If clinical suspicion is high, further testing is needed regardless of the findings on the first endoscopy.

The first step in making an accurate assessment of oropharyngeal dysphagia is screening. In the document "Preferred Practice Patterns for the Profession of Speech-Language Pathology," the American Speech-Language-Hearing Association (ASHA) defines dysphagia screening as "a pass/fail procedure to identify individuals who require a comprehensive assessment of swallowing function or a referral for other professional and/or medical services."[4] Screening is typically performed by the SLP in the office or by other allied health care providers such as nurses in the hospital setting. The individual being screened is deemed to be either at risk or not at risk for oropharyngeal dysphagia.

Screening tools are meant to be quick and efficient, and to save time and money by identifying individuals who are at risk for dysphagia and aspiration and who may require further assessment. A screening allows the clinician to identify individuals who truly need a full, more expensive and time-consuming evaluation and prevents unnecessary utilization of these resources for individuals who do not.

Many approaches to screening have been suggested. Some suggest a screen should include a question-only approach. Although it was originally intended as an outcomes tool, there is evidence that the Eating Assessment Tool (EAT-10)[5] can be used as a tool for predicting aspiration risk.[6–8] Other approaches to screening include presentation of one or more boluses. What those boluses are and what bolus volumes are included differ. Many screenings incorporate water swallow tests,[9–13] although bolus size varies among the different water screenings. Some utilize up to 10 small boluses of 3 to 5 mL of water,[9,14,15] while others incorporate larger volumes of water of as much as 90 to 100 mL.[10–13] A recent systemic review and meta-analysis of screening methods that incorporated a water swallow test revealed high specificity but low sensitivity for small bolus volumes, whereas water swallow tests incorporating consecutive sips of larger bolus volumes (90–100 mL) demonstrated higher sensitivity but lower specificity.[16] In clinical practice and due to higher sensitivity, the large bolus screening appears to be a better screening tool through which people who actually have aspiration do not go undetected.

If a patient passes a valid, reliable, sensitive screen, a full swallowing evaluation, such as an instrumental assessment of swallowing (ie, modified barium swallow), is not needed and the patient is safe to begin receiving medications, liquids, and food without the need for further assessment.

A failed screening indicates further assessment is needed. In the case of dysphagia, a patient who fails a valid and reliable screening should be referred to an SLP for further assessment.

CLINICAL SWALLOW EVALUATION

The clinical swallow evaluation (CSE) is often the next level of evaluation in the assessment of individuals at risk for oropharyngeal dysphagia. According to ASHA,[17] the CSE allows the SLP to:

- Integrate information from interview/case history, review medical records, and make observations from a physical exam
- Observe and assess integrity and function of the structures in the upper airway and digestive tract
- Identify the presence of and observe the characteristics of dysphagia based on clinical signs and symptoms
- Identify clinical signs and symptoms of esophageal dysphagia or gastroesophageal reflux disease (GERD)
- Determine the need for an instrumental exam (more objective assessment of swallow)
- Determine if the patient is an appropriate candidate for treatment and/or management
- Recommend an appropriate route of nutritional management
- Recommend clinical interventions

Indications for a Clinical Swallow Evaluation

It is important for the SLP to understand what prompted the referral for a CSE and what the referring provider's primary concern is regarding the patient. If a screening has been administered, failure results in referral for clinical or instrumental assessment. In other cases, the physician may refer directly to the SLP without the patient completing a prior screening. Referral for a CSE may be based upon the patient's medical diagnosis or the patient's nutritional status.

Often the patient's complaints prompt the physician referral to an SLP for a CSE. Patients may complain of frequent coughing or choking during meals, feeling as if food or liquid gets stuck when they attempt to swallow, or prolonged meal times. They may also complain of pain associated with swallowing, odynophagia, or food or liquid coming out of their nose when they attempt to swallow. Any of these complaints may indicate an underlying swallowing problem and should result in referral for a CSE.

Components of the Clinical Swallow Evaluation

Chart Review

The first step in the evaluation is a thorough chart review. The chart review assists the clinician in formulating a hypothesis regarding the nature of the patient's swallowing difficulty.

In the case of patients with chronic cough, it is particularly important to note any current or previous illnesses that correspond with onset of dysphagia symptoms, such as a recent upper respiratory infection. If the patient has a history of frequent upper respiratory illness, chronic aspiration should be considered as a possible cause. Presence of pneumonia or a history of pneumonia are highly predictive of aspiration risk.[17] History of upper respiratory infection or respiratory failure necessitating intubation or tracheotomy should be noted. Repeated intubations or extubations, or traumatic intubations or extubations, can lead to laryngeal irritation or vocal fold motion impairment, with chronic cough occurring as a result of aspiration or penetration in the face of glottic incompetence. Additionally, clinicians should note whether the patient has a history of gastroesophageal reflux and if the patient is on medications to control reflux symptoms. Laryngopharyngeal reflux (LPR) can result in irritation to the larynx and hypopharynx and, more importantly, is postulated to cause protective upper esophageal sphincter hyperfunction that results in a feeling of difficulty swallowing. LPR is discussed in detail in Chapter 4.

Surgical history should also be reviewed. Specifically, previous surgery to the head and neck, including tracheostomy or surgical resection of head and neck cancer, should be noted. Surgeries can result in anatomical alterations that lead to changes in swallow physiology. Previous history of feeding tube placement may indicate a history of dysphagia or malnutrition.

The chart review should also include a review of current medications. Certain medications can adversely affect swallow function, either as a normal side effect of the drug or as a complication of the therapeutic action of the drug.[18,19] Medications that affect smooth or striated esophageal muscle function may cause dysphagia. Dysphagia resulting from a complication of the therapeutic action of a medication includes viral or fungal esophagitis in patients treated with immunosuppressive drugs or cancer therapeutic agents, or medications that can depress the central nervous system, such as benzodiazepines. Additionally, some medications such as nonsteroidal anti-inflammatory drugs (NSAIDS) can cause esophagitis, stricture formation, or esophageal ulceration with chronic use, leading to dysphagia symptoms.[20] Other medications may cause xerostomia (dry mouth) and interfere with oral transit of the bolus, result in laryngeal irritation, particulate retention, and lead to chronic cough. Clinicians should also note if patients have been prescribed angiotensin-converting enzyme inhibitors (ACE inhibitors), as chronic cough may occur as a side effect in up to 10% of individuals taking these medications, and occurs more frequently in women than in men.[21]

Case History

The next step in clinical assessment is a thorough case history. The aim of the case history is to assist the clinician in formulating a hypothesis regarding the underlying pathophysiology causing the patient's symptoms. The information gathered during the case history can be invaluable in determining the appropriate means of assessing swallowing function, for instance fluoroscopy or endoscopy, and in determining whether other professions, such as gastroenterology or neurology, should be consulted.

Chief Complaint

Common patient complaints include coughing, choking or strangling with food or liquids, food or liquids sticking in the throat, difficulty chewing, and prolonged mealtimes. In a patient with a history of chronic cough, it is particularly important to ask if coughing increases during or after eating or drinking. Increased coughing during eating can indicate penetration or aspiration of food or liquid; increased coughing after meals can indicate reflux, esophageal dysmotility, or a cervical diverticulum. Additionally, patient complaints of feeling as if food sticks, difficulty swallowing solid foods (often breads or steak), or difficulty swallowing liquids of extreme temperatures (either hot or cold) may indicate an esophageal phase issue rather than an oropharyngeal swallowing difficulty.[22]

History of Symptoms

Clinicians should also ask patients about the timeline of their dysphagia. Questions should include duration of dysphagia symptoms, whether the patient experienced any illnesses at the time dysphagia symptoms began, and if symptoms vary depending upon time of day. Patients reporting symptoms that are worse upon awakening and/or shortly thereafter may be experiencing gastroesophageal reflux, whereas those reporting a progression of their symptoms throughout the day or throughout the course of a meal may be experiencing muscle weakness or fatigue related to an underlying neurological condition. Changes in vocal quality that accompany the onset of the patient's dysphagia can point to vocal fold pathology and warrant a closer look with laryngovideostroboscopy. For example, oropharyngeal sensation issues that lead to hypopharyngeal pooling and spill over into the larynx with a resultant "wet" sounding voice.

Oral Mechanism Examination

Another critical component of the CSE is the oral mechanism examination. Integrity of the lips, tongue, face, hard and soft palate, dentition, oral health, and jaw should be assessed at rest and during functional movement. The oral mechanism examination can help the clinician form hypotheses regarding the nature of the patient's swallowing disorder. The oral mechanism examination provides a means of assessing the integrity of the cranial nerves involved in swallowing and may indicate which aspects of swallow function are impaired. The cranial nerves involved in swallowing are the trigeminal (V), facial (VII), glossopharyngeal (IX), vagus (X), and hypoglossal (XII).

In patients with chronic cough, assessment of vagal nerve function is particularly important. The glossopharyngeal nerve and the vagus nerve are often damaged together. Thus, integrity of these nerves can be assessed simultaneously. Clinicians should observe the velum (soft palate) at rest and during elevation (ie, while saying "Ah"). Vocal quality can indicate functionality of these nerves. Breathy vocal quality may indicate unilateral or bilateral vocal fold dysfunction that places the patient at increased risk for aspiration due to decreased airway protection during swallowing. There are a number of studies indicating the presence of dysphonia, including breathiness, harshness, or hoarseness, is predictive of aspiration.[23,24] Others have suggested reduced pitch elevation is predictive of dysphagia due to co-existing sensation issues associated with a superior laryngeal neuropaty.[25] Clinicians may also want to elicit a gag response from their patients to assess integrity of CNs IX and X. Integrity of the patient's voluntary cough can be used to assess glossopharyngeal and vagus nerve function. Objective measures of voluntary cough, using tools such as a pneumotachograph, have high sensitivity and specificity for detecting aspiration risk.[26] Smith-Hammond found significant reductions in peak expiratory airflow in patients with dysphagia following stroke. Individuals with severe aspiration exhibited the lowest peak expiratory airflows during a voluntary cough.[27] Additionally, peak expiratory flow rates are reduced in patients with Parkinson's disease who aspirate compared to those who do not aspirate.[28,29] Finally, cough peak flow can be used to predict pulmonary complications resulting from aspiration in individuals with dysphagia.[30]

One method of assessing integrity of the cough reflex is cough reflex testing, in which the patient is asked to actively or passively inhale a solution containing either tartaric acid, citric acid, or capsaicin. Integrity of either a natural cough response or a suppressed cough response is assessed. Abnormal or reduced cough response following inhalation of these solutions has been found to predict risk of pneumonia in individuals with stroke in some studies but not in others.[31–35]

Bolus Administration

When administering a CSE, a standardized protocol of bolus administration is recommended. Standardization of bolus types, numbers of boluses, and bolus amounts allows for comparison of patient behavior across trials. Additionally, it ensures consistency across clinicians and across facilities. Typically, a CSE will include presentation of a thin liquid (often water), a pureed or pudding-type bolus, and a solid consistency. Boluses of each may be presented in varying amounts, often progressing from very small amounts and progressing to larger amounts that are considered to be more reflective of typical patient behavior (eg, cup sips of thin liquids or self-fed pudding or solid boluses). Patients are observed for any signs/symptoms of oropharyngeal dysphagia.

Oral phase issues that may be observed include reduced lip seal resulting in spillage of the bolus from the oral cavity, inefficient or ineffective mastication of solid textures, and residue within the oral cavity. Little information about integrity of the pharyngeal phase of swallowing can be gleaned from the CSE. Structures in the pharynx, such as the base of tongue, posterior pharyngeal wall, valleculae, and pyriform sinuses, cannot be visualized without the aid of instrumentation such as an endoscope or X-ray. On the other hand, signs and symptoms of aspiration can be detected during a CSE. Cough is one of the most reliable signs of aspiration.[26,27,38] Wet vocal quality immediately post-swallow has also been suggested to have predictive value for detecting aspiration.[23,38] However, clinicians do not reliably perceive wet vocal quality when material is present in the larynx during phonation, and judgment of vocal quality lacks sensitivity and specificity for detection of aspiration.[39,40] Thus, clinicians should consider referring for or performing videostroboscopy if the voice is abnormal but should be cautious in making judgments of aspiration risk based solely on changes in vocal quality. The likelihood that a patient is going to present with overt signs/symptoms of aspiration appears to be dependent on bolus volume. Presentation of small bolus volumes of 1 to 5 mL lack sufficient sensitivity for detection of aspiration, and patients who aspirate silently may not be identified if only small bolus volumes are presented. Larger bolus volumes of 90 to 100 mL have high sensitivity for detection of aspiration, and patients who aspirate silently when presented with small bolus volumes are less likely to do so when they take larger bolus volumes.[40,41] Despite the ease of use and clinical utility of the CSE, a recent review paper showed that the sensitivity and specificity of water swallow tests compared to the standard of radiographic or endoscopic imaging was 71% and 90%, respectively, for single sip volumes, 91% and 53% for consecutive 90 to 100 mL trials, and 86% and 65% for progressively increasing volumes of water.[41]

INSTRUMENTATION

Next Steps

If the patient exhibits no overt signs or symptoms of aspiration or dysphagia, and if the patient is medically stable, the clinician may wish to recommend an oral diet. If overt signs or symptoms of aspiration or dysphagia were observed during the CSE, an instrumental assessment such as videofluoroscopy or endoscopy is recommended.

Videofluoroscopy

The videofluoroscopic swallow study (VFSS), also called the modified barium swallow (MBS), is a radiographic procedure during which swallowing is viewed in real time. It is considered the criterion standard for evaluating the oral, pharyngeal, and cervical esophageal phases of swallowing. The purpose of the VFSS is to determine underlying swallow pathophysiology resulting in the patient's symptoms of dysphagia and to determine appropriate treatment options. Patients are given a series of barium sulfate-infused boluses, ranging from thin liquid to solid, and swallowing is observed in the lateral and anterior-posterior views. As with the CSE, a standardized protocol is recommended. Because videofluoroscopy is a radiographic procedure, it is a time-limited examination. Fluoroscopy time is typically limited to 5 minutes or less.

During the VFSS, structural movements including tongue movement, velar elevation, hyoid superior and anterior movement, laryngeal elevation, epiglottic retroflexion, base of tongue retraction, pharyngoesophageal segment opening, and pharyngeal stripping wave are observed. Additionally, timing of swallowing events, including oral transit times, initiation of the pharyngeal swallow, pharyngeal transit times, and duration of cricopharyngeal opening are viewed. Clinicians should note presence of residual material in various locations including the lateral sulci, base of tongue, posterior pharyngeal wall, valleculae, and pyriform sinuses as well as the patient's response to the residue. In some instances, very small amounts of residual material remaining in the pharynx after the swallow will create a sufficient irritant to elicit the patient's urge to cough or clear his or her throat. Penetration, defined as liquid or food entering the laryngeal vestibule but not spilling below the vocal folds, and/or aspiration, defined as liquid or food spilling below the vocal folds, should be noted as should the underlying pathophysiologic problem that led to the finding. Again, the patient's response or lack thereof to penetration or aspiration should be reported. Of particular importance is whether the patient responds with cough or throat clear to aspiration, an event known as "silent aspiration" when there is no response.

One common finding on the VFSS is the presence of a cricopharyngeal (CP) bar at the pharyngoesophageal segment. A CP bar is defined as an unremitting prominence of the CP muscle during a swallow when it should relax as seen in lateral view on radiographic imaging (Figure 7–1). The CP bar is thought to be significant when it occludes more than 50% of the lumen when filled with contrast and relates to its reduction of maximal dimensions of the upper esophageal sphincter (UES), causing presumed increased intrabolus pressure upstream to the UES.[42]

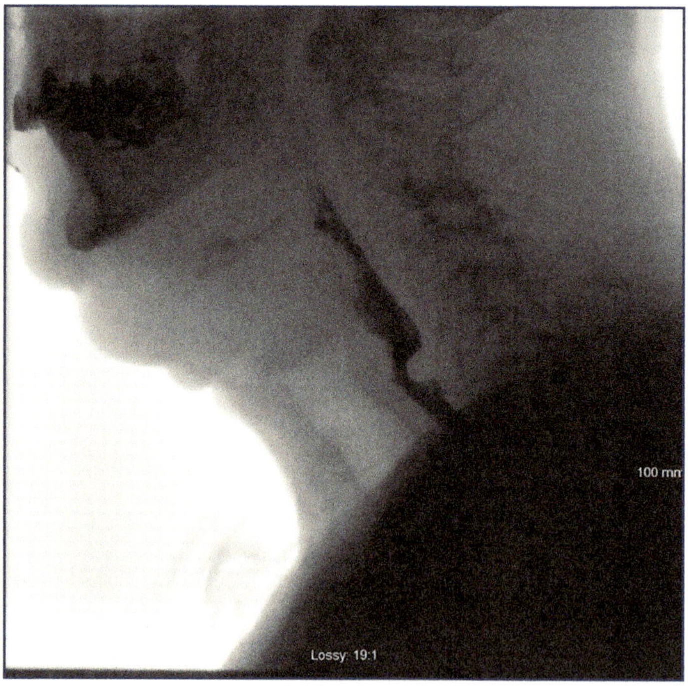

Figure 7–1. VFSS view of a cricopharyngeal bar in an individual after radiation treatment for head and neck cancer.

Flexible Endoscopic Evaluation of Swallowing (FEES)

Flexible Endoscopic Evaluation of Swallowing (FEES) was introduced in the 1980s as an adjunct to the VFSS. It involves the transnasal passage of a flexible fiberoptic or distal chip endoscope into the oropharynx to allow for a superior view of the structures of the pharynx and the larynx. Structures of the hypopharynx and endolarynx are observed prior to and following the pharyngeal phase of swallowing. Because the endoscope is placed through the nasal cavity, the oral phase cannot be viewed. During onset of the pharyngeal swallow, the tip of the endoscope is deflected when the base of tongue contacts the posterior pharyngeal wall. This period, known as "white-out," typically lasts less than 0.5 seconds. Structures can then be observed following completion of the pharyngeal phase.

Prior to placing the endoscope, clinicians may wish to administer a topical anesthetic such as viscous lidocaine and/or a vasoconstrictor such as oxymetazoline (Afrin) to enhance patient comfort during the examination. Clinicians should take care to ensure that the anesthetic is administered to the tip of the nose rather than more posteriorly as there is the potential for the anesthetic to enter the pharynx. Swallow function may be affected adversely if this occurs. Anesthesia can impact swallow function negatively by altering the normal timing of bolus flow and decreasing sensitivity to penetrated or aspirated material.[43,44] In patients with chronic cough, it is particularly undesirable to anesthetize the laryngopharynx because the clinician wishes to observe any patient reaction to scope placement, residue, or penetration/aspiration. Many patients are able to tolerate endoscope placement without the need for topical anesthetic or vasoconstrictor.[45]

A typical FEES begins with observation of velopharyngeal function. Patients repeat a series of syllables containing nasal phonemes (/n/, /m/, /ng/) and non-nasal phonemes (any vowel or any other consonant). Adequacy of and pattern of velopharyngeal closure are noted. The endoscopist then advances the tip of the endoscope into the oropharynx. Here, the endoscope visualizes the structures of the larynx and hypopharynx including the base of tongue, posterior pharyngeal wall, epiglottis, valleculae, pyriform sinuses, aryepiglottic folds, laryngeal vestibule, false vocal folds, true vocal folds, subglottis, and the superior trachea. It is important to note the presence and location of any secretions. Before any foods or liquids are presented to the patient, the presence of secretions in the endolarynx indicates an increased likelihood of thin liquid aspiration and reduced laryngeal sensation.[46,47] Clinicians may also observe the patient aspirating secretions. This is unobservable during a VFSS. Should aspiration of secretions be observed, clinicians may opt not to provide any boluses to the patient during the examination.

Assessment of pharyngeal and supraglottic laryngeal sensation, and thus, integrity of the superior laryngeal nerve and airway protection, has been suggested as an adjunct to the traditional endoscopic evaluation of swallowing.[48–50] Fiberoptic endoscopic evaluation of swallowing with sensory testing (FEESST) was introduced in the 1990s.[49,50] Using a special two-channel flexible endoscope, an air puff is delivered to the aryepiglottic folds, eliciting the laryngeal adductor response (LAR). Absence of the LAR is considered a sign of increased risk of silent aspiration during the subsequent swallow examination. Normative values for threshold responses to the air puff are lacking, and the specialized equipment necessary to perform FEESST is no longer commercially available. In lieu of FEESST, clinicians may apply light pressure to the mucosa over the bilateral arytenoid cartilages to assess integrity of laryngeal sensation. An intact response is indicated by a white-out response on endoscopy.[51] Although this method was not found to be sensitive to minor sensory deficits, it was found to identify more severe sensory problems accurately.[52] In practice, a lack of any response to light touch with the tip of the endoscope is evidence of decreased sensation.

Following inspection of the pharyngeal and laryngeal structures, swallowing is assessed. Swallow function is observed prior to onset and after completion of the pharyngeal phase of swallowing. Typically, the patient self-feeds or is given a series of boluses that can range from ice chips to solid textures. In some instances, such as when there is a significant concern for medical stability should the patient aspirate on food or liquid during the examination, the clinician may choose not to administer any boluses. FEES testing offers a distinct advantage over a VFSS because, if the clinician chooses, no boluses need be administered.

If the clinician opts to present liquid or food during the evaluation, boluses are often dyed with blue or green food coloring to enhance visualization during the examination. However, use of opaque substances such as milk or vanilla pudding generally allows for adequate visualization.[53] A standardized protocol of bolus administration is generally advised, as it allows for comparison of function across examinations in order to determine patient change across examination sessions. Often, thin liquids are presented first if there is not already a strong suspicion for an aspiration risk. Other bolus types that may be presented during the examination include a pudding or pureed texture as well as a solid texture, such as a shortbread cookie or graham cracker.

Transnasal Esophagoscopy

Sometimes the VFSS or FEES does not explain the cough symptoms despite a good patient history for dysphagia and further information is needed. The reason for the cough may arise from further down in the esophagus due to the vagal reflex mechanism or other esophageal pathology. Transnasal esophagoscopy (TNE) is a tool that allows the clinician to easily visualize the esophagus, lower esophageal sphincter, and stomach in awake, unsedated patients to evaluate for reflux, globus, dysphagia, and head and neck cancer.[54] TNE has been reported to show significant findings in 50% of procedures performed.[55] These findings include esophagitis, hiatal hernia, Barrett's esophagus, candidiasis, stricture, carcinoma, abnormal motility, esophageal webs, and esophageal diverticula. The otolaryngologist may be ideally suited to screen for mucosal changes in the esophagus because researchers have found that those patients with Barrett's esophagus have a higher prevalence of LPR symptoms, especially chronic cough, than typical GERD symptoms.[56] In a recent study, Howell furthermore showed that 51% of patients undergoing TNE had a finding that resulted in a change in management such as an esophageal stricture, irregular z-line, reflux esophagitis, or infectious esophagitis.[57] This incidence of esophageal findings was even higher in those patients with elevated EAT-10 scores or a history of head and neck cancer (81% if both head and neck cancer with dysphagia history).

TNE is performed in the office with no sedation. First, a topical oxymetazoline and 4% lidocaine mixture is sprayed into the nose and then cottonoids soaked with the same mixture are placed into the bilateral nares for 5 to 10 minutes. It should be noted that if the patient was unable to tolerate the regular flexible laryngoscope, they will be unlikely able to tolerate the slightly larger diameter of the TNE scope (it contains a working channel and is thus wider). No further anesthesia is used in the laryngopharynx as it has been found previously to make patients gag, aspirate, and generally be more uncomfortable than when just having the scope inside. The scope is advanced through the naris that appears more spacious, preferably through an inferior route between the inferior turbinate, nasal septum, and floor of nose, and then passed into the hypopharynx and directed above the cleft between the posterior cricoid and the posterior oropharyngeal wall. The patient is directed to swallow at this point and then the practitioner advances the scope gently until reaching the stomach. No forceful move should be undertaken, and the lumen should be kept in view, but visualization is easier when pulling the scope back out as it centers the scope. The stomach is viewed and then the scope is retroflexed (turned 180 degrees back on itself) to allow a view of the scope as it passes through the lower esophageal sphincter (LES), which affords a view of the strength (or patency) of the lower esophageal sphincter around the scope as well as the passage of saliva when the patient swallows. Air is then sucked out of the stomach and the z-line is identified, the junction where the squamous mucosa of the esophagus and the columnar mucosa of the esophagus meet. Figure 7–2 shows a typical view of the gastroesophageal z-line. The anatomic gastroesophageal junction (GEJ) is an area that represents the junction between the distal esophagus and the proximal stomach or cardia and the most proximal aspect of the gastric folds.[58] In this area of the LES, the diaphragmatic pinch occurs where the diaphragm squeezes

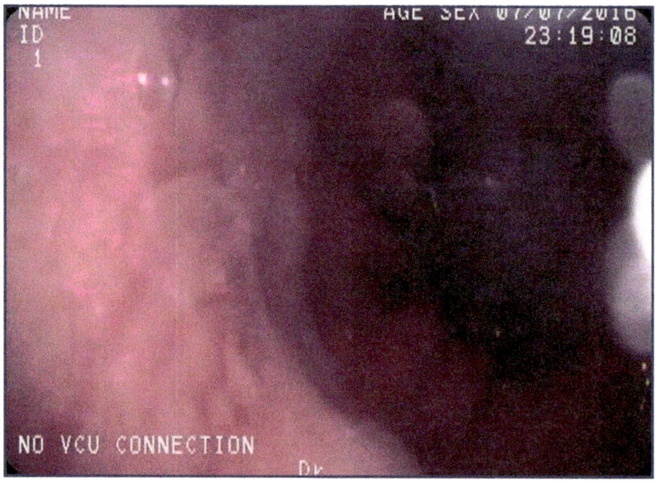

Figure 7–2. TNE view of the z-line where the esophageal mucosa transitions to gastric mucosa. It is perturbations of this area and extension of ulcerations that should prompt biopsies to rule out Barrett's esophagus and other pathologies.

around the esophagus as it passes through it and out of the thoracic cavity. Further anatomic pathology such as a hiatal hernia can be identified here, where the gastric rugae push up through the diaphragm into the thoracic cavity, distorting the usual relationship of the LES and the diaphragm. Any other distortion of the usual z-line should be biopsied, as this could represent Barrett's esophagus (where the normal tissue lining of the esophagus is replaced with lining that resembles the intestine) which is only proven pathologically. Barrett's esophagus is thought to be a complication of chronic GERD and a precursor lesion in most cases of esophageal adenocarcinoma.[59] As compared to a general Danish population, the relative risk of adenocarcinoma in patients with Barrett's esophagus was 11.3%.[60] Detection of low-grade dysplasia on biopsy was an even greater relative risk. Further biopsies can be undertaken in the lower and/or mid esophagus to rule out eosinophilic esophagitis if this is being considered for the patient. Biopsies are not generally painful or even appreciated by the patient in the mid to lower esophagus, but often become more uncomfortable the closer the biopsy is taken to the pharynx. Delivering small puffs of air to keep the esophagus dilated to view all mucosal surfaces or spraying water to remove any food debris on the scope or on the esophageal wall is helpful at intervals to allow better visualization. When evaluating the esophagus, asking the patient to swallow occasionally can also improve the view without the need for as much insufflation, which can lead to a sensation of bloating for some patients. The whole exam should be recorded to allow review by the clinician and with the patient.

High-Resolution Esophageal Manometry

High-resolution esophageal manometry (HRM) is a tool used to investigate esophageal symptoms after mechanical obstruction and mucosal disease have been excluded by endoscopy or radiographic examinations.[61] Impedance monitoring, sometimes performed simultaneously with HRM, increases the diagnostic yield for evaluating potential gastroesophageal, gastropharyngeal (LPR) or esophagopharyngeal (liquid originating from esophageal dysmotility and not from the stomach) reflux disease.[62] HRM is further useful in its ability to classify esophageal disorders more specifically in those with nonobstructive dysphagia. Future uses of the same technology to assess pharyngeal muscle weakness ("pharyngeal manometry") are in their infancy but gaining popularity.

Technology has allowed a movement from water-perfused HRM systems to more solid-state systems and for the spacing to be shrunk to approximately 1 cm between sensors to allow for higher resolution.[63] Computer technology has also afforded the processing of the large amount of data generated that is then used to develop line plots into spatiotemporal plots. More information on HRM is presented in Chapter 4.

DYSPHAGIA PATHOLOGIES AND COUGH

This chapter has focused on the diagnostic and clinical tools the clinician can use to diagnose swallowing problems that can lead to aspiration or abnormalities in the swallow that can lead to cough. In this section, specific swallowing abnormalities and how they are associated with cough will be addressed.

Zenker's Diverticulum

Cough can be one of the most common presenting symptoms of a Zenker's or another cervical diverticulum. In the case of a Zenker's diverticulum, outpouching of the esophageal wall through Killian's dehiscence between the inferior pharyngeal constrictor and the cricopharyngeus will sometimes serve as a fluid or food reservoir that can empty back into the throat and cause delayed coughing after the swallow. This delay is important, as coughing with thin liquids immediately after swallowing is a warning sign for an unsafe swallow, as illustrated earlier. Diverticula of the esophagus should be easily visualized with the VFSS. Figure 7–3 shows a Zenker's diverticulum on lateral view with contrast retained within it. Wirth and

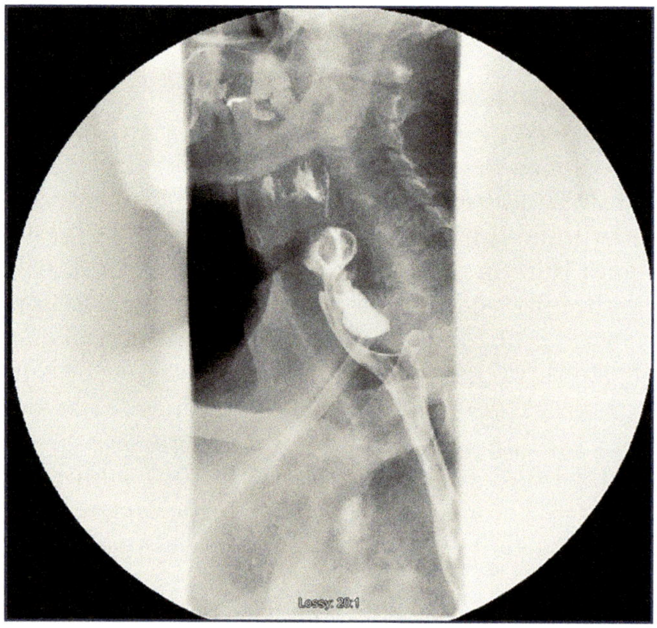

Figure 7–3. VFSS lateral view of a Zenker's diverticulum retaining barium contrast within it.

colleagues showed that patients had symptoms of dysphagia (96%), regurgitation (60%), and cough (19%), followed by pneumonia (9%) in patients with Zenker's.[64] Most patients get relief from their coughing after their pouch is treated in a surgical fashion that disrupts the CP muscle, allowing the pouch to empty and avoid subsequent regurgitation into and irritation of the larynx. In the same study, no instances of aspiration pneumonia were found in postoperative patients regardless of surgical approach (endoscopic CP myotomy or via an open resection and CP myotomy).

Foreign Body

Dysphagia may be a predisposing factor for aerodigestive foreign bodies. A complete food impaction in the esophagus could provide very significant pooling in the pharynx that could lead to aspiration and cough as a protective measure. Alternatively, dysphagia and incoordination of the pharyngeal swallow could more readily lead to airway foreign bodies.[65] Airway foreign bodies are often very evident when they are occurring due to a robust cough and potential stridor or dyspnea. Less commonly, a person or child will not recognize a foreign body aspiration event, and eventually an infection will develop distal to the foreign body in the airways and a subsequent cough will develop.[66]

Eosinophilic Esophagitis

Eosinophilic esophagitis (EoE) is characterized by the clinical findings of food impaction and dysphagia in adults, but in children the symptoms are less severe, such as feeding intolerance and symptoms consistent with GERD.[67] Importantly, patients frequently have symptoms such as coughing or dysphonia in their initial presentations. The key histological finding in EoE is eosinophilic infiltration of the esophageal mucosa with more than 15 intraepithelial eosinophils per high-power field in one or more biopsies. A dense esophageal eosinophilia is often described in association with severe squamous epithelial hyperplasia. There is a strong correlation between EoE, atopy, aeroallergen polysensitization, and food allergens.[68] Additionally, Kelly et al, showed that an elemental diet improved clinical and histologic findings in 10 children with EoE.[69] Importantly, and not always clearly distinguishable, GERD is supposed to be absent before EoE can be accurately diagnosed.

It is important for the clinician to be aware of EoE because it is the primary cause of dysphagia and esophageal impaction in children and young adults and the second most common cause of esophagitis after GERD, and has similar symptoms to GERD and LPR, especially in those patients who do not respond to proton-pump inhibitors.[70] TNE with esophageal biopsies is effective at obtaining tissue specimens to confirm the diagnosis of EoE or rule it out.

Reflux

While GERD is covered more at length in Chapter 4 of this book, we will briefly mention it here, as it is considered to be one of the most common causes of chronic cough and dysphagia. Mechanisms that have been postulated include direct stimulation within the esophageal mucosa of the nerve terminals responsible for evoking cough either in the larynx or bronchi via indirect stimulation of neural pathways linking the esophagus to the airway (the bronchoesophageal reflex).[71] Current evidence is scant in support of direct provocation of coughing by refluxate in the laryngopharynx, and it is more common for patients to have a reflux-related cough that does not necessarily correlate with a specific reflux event of impedance testing. Only 20% to 48% of patients have a positive symptom association probability for reflux events preceding cough, assuming a link if these events happen within 5 minutes of one another.[71] As noted in Chapter 5, because of the likely prominent role the digestive enzyme pepsin plays in the pathophysiology of LPR symptoms such as cough, future strategies to treat cough-associated reflux will likely include treatments that decrease the number of reflux events, not just decrease the acidity or treat the underlying pepsin itself.

Conversely, cough itself does not seem to cause a reflux event into the laryngopharynx. HRM has shown that a cough induces a rise in the UES pressure, raising it significantly higher than in the esophagus, lower esophageal sphincter, and stomach.[72] This suggests that a cough could increase reflux from the stomach into the esophagus and, in those prone to coughing, could set them up for a subsequent LPR event after the cough or trigger the abovementioned bronchoesophageal cough reflex.

Achalasia

Achalasia is a primary esophageal motor disorder of unknown etiology affecting all genders and all ages. It affects roughly 0.5 to 1 per 100,000 people in the United States.[73] It is defined by an absence of normal peristalsis and failure of relaxation of the LES as demonstrated on esophageal manometry. Sinan and colleagues looked at a cohort of 110 patients presenting with achalasia to one center.[74] Not surprisingly, 86% of these patients complained of dysphagia at least daily. However, 37% reported cough and 31% had aspiration symptoms. All told, 40% of patients had at least one respiratory symptom. They then looked at a subgroup of 22 patients who had manometry before and after a Heller myotomy (cutting of the lower esophageal sphincter muscles) for treatment of the achalasia. They found that cough was improved in eight out of 10 patients postoperatively, and aspiration was improved in 10 out of 11 patients. A case report of a patient presenting with chronic cough who had previously failed conventional GERD treatment achieved cough resolution after pneumatic dilation to treat her achalasia.[75]

Gupta et al looked at pulmonary function before and after pneumatic dilation for achalasia.[76] Spirometry showed abnormalities in 45% of patients prior to treatment. They found significant improvements in forced expiratory ventilation in 1 second (FEV_1), forced vital capacity (FVC), peak expiratory flow rate (PEFR), and midexpiratory flow rate ($MEF_{25\text{-}75}$) in postop spirometry performed a month after dilation. The balloon they used to dilate was 30 mm in diameter in females and 35 mm in males. The fact that patients experienced an improvement in their cough after dilation of their LES suggests a possible causal relationship between achalasia and cough.

Aging

The majority of chronic cough patients attending specialist clinics are middle-aged or elderly persons,[77] and cough is also reportedly one of the most frequent problems for which people present for medical care.[78]

Older patients (>65 or >70, depending on the study) have higher rates of disordered swallowing and other feeding problems.[79,80] More specifically, older patients have been found to have decreased peristaltic response to wet swallows when compared to younger patients.[81,82] Decreased contraction amplitude, polyphasic esophageal contractions, esophageal dilatation and decreased sphincter relaxations have also been reported in older individuals.[83–86] Direct contribution from aging is difficult to pin down because other comorbid conditions accompany increased age and thereby confounds causation. However, a recent study looked at esophageal motor function in older and younger asymptomatic healthy adults. They found subtle changes in the LES with a trend toward a lower basal LES pressure and a reduction of complete LES relaxation.[87] It is also suggested that after a lifetime of UES hyperfunction to protect the laryngopharynx from reflux, the pharyngeal muscles become less effective over time from pushing against the hypertensive CP muscle. This is potentially reversible with CP myotomy.[88]

Other Conditions

There are several other conditions that are related to both cough and dysphagia. Progressive systemic sclerosis, or scleroderma, is a chronic autoimmune disease characterized by proliferative lesions with resultant fibrosis of skin and multiple organs, including the gastrointestinal tract and the lungs.[89] Upper or lower gastrointestinal (GI) involvement is reported in up to 90% of patients with scleroderma. GI involvement generally occurs as a spectrum of problems with motility and transit time from asymptomatic to severe paresis anywhere along the GI tract, including esophageal dysmotility. Cough has also been found in several patients with interstitial lung disease due to scleroderma. There is circumstantial evidence that neurogenic inflammation may be involved in lung fibrosis and cough.[90] These patients have several different potential or contributing causes to their coughs due to the often concomitant problems of esophageal dysmotility and gastroesophageal reflux.

There has also been association of cough with jackhammer esophagus.[91] Jackhammer esophagus is a major motility abnormality characterized on HRM as at least 20% of liquid swallows having a distal contractile integral greater than 8000 mm Hg/s/cm. In one study that included 17 patients who met strict criteria, 29% had noncardiac chest pain, 47% had dysphagia, and 24% had other symptoms such as cough, heartburn, or regurgitation.

THINKING OUTSIDE OF THE BOX

Every patient who presents with a cough complaint is different. Dysphagia should be screened with a minimum of two key questions: "Do you have to avoid any certain foods?" or "Do you cough or choke on liquids when you swallow?" Further testing should be warranted if patients answer yes to any of these questions or your clinical suspicion is high. Additionally, if all other tests and treatments have been attempted and the patient is still seeking medical care for their chronic cough, it behooves the provider to be thorough with a dysphagia assessment to rule out this overlooked etiology.

Most exciting in the evaluation and treatment of patients with oropharyngeal and pharyngoesophageal dysphagia is the advent of one high-resolution pharyngeal manometry (HRPM). O'Rourke and Humphries recently published on their use of HRPM in a patient to provide biofeedback.[92] Their patient had a VFSS showing poor airway protection and pharyngeal clearance along with residue in the postcricoid region consistent with cricopharyngeal dysfunction. HRPM was able to show normal relaxation of the upper esophageal sphincter, including both opening and relaxation pressures, thus directing treatment away from cricopharyngeus muscle surgery. In this case, HRPM was able to show an absence of inferior constrictor contractility, which could be addressed nonsurgically via weekly biofeedback sessions with HRPM and swallowing exercises. This allowed effective symptom improvement and demonstrates the potential for this newer advancement in the use of HRM as an adjunct to diagnosis and therapy for swallowing disorders.

TAKE-HOME POINTS

- Dysphagia and aspiration should always be considered when patients present with a chronic cough.
- There are many reasons why liquids, solids, and saliva elicit a cough reflex in the pharynx and esophagus. Some are protective in nature, while some are pathologic and unnecessary from an airway protection standpoint.
- There is clearly a continuum of appropriate cough reflexes that are appropriate for protecting the airway, but inadequate airway protection or unnecessary coughing leads patients to seek medical attention.
- Having a fundamental grasp on the tools that can assess the oral cavity, pharynx, larynx, and esophagus during swallowing is necessary to fully assess and treat cough patients.

REFERENCES

1. Amin MR, Koufman JA. Vagal neuropathy after upper respiratory infection: a viral etiology? *Am J Otolaryngol.* 2001;22(4):251–256.
2. Rees CJ, Henderson AH, Belafsky PC. Postviral vagal neuropathy. *Ann Otol Rhinol Laryngol.* 2009;118(4):247–252.
3. Achilleos A. Evidence-based evaluation and management of chronic cough. *Med Clin North Am.* 2016;100(5):1033–1045.
4. American Speech-Language-Hearing Association. Preferred practice patterns for the profession of speech-language pathology. 2004.
5. Belafsky PC, Mouadeb DA, Rees CJ, et al. Validity and reliability of the Eating Assessment Tool (EAT-10). *Ann Otol Rhinol Laryngol.* 2008;117(12):919–924.
6. Arslan SS, Demir N, Kilinc HE, Karaduman AA. The ability of the Eating Assessment Tool-10 to detect aspiration in patients with neurological disorders. *J Neurogastroenterol Motil.* 2017;23(4):550–554.
7. Cheney DM, Siddiqui MT, Litts JK, Kuhn MA, Belafsky PC. The ability of the 10-Item Eating Assessment Tool (EAT-10) to predict aspiration risk in persons with dysphagia. *Ann Otol Rhinol Laryngol.* 2015;124(5):351–354.
8. Plowman EK, Tabor LC, Robison R, et al. Discriminant ability of the Eating Assessment Tool-10 to detect aspiration in individuals with amyotrophic lateral sclerosis. *Neurogastroenterol Motil.* 2016;28(1):85–90.
9. Martino R, Silver F, Teasell R, et al. The Toronto Bedside Swallowing Screening Test (TOR-BSST): development and validation of a dysphagia screening tool for patients with stroke. *Stroke.* 2009;40(2):555–561.
10. Suiter DM, Sloggy J, Leder SB. Validation of the Yale Swallow Protocol: a prospective double-blinded videofluoroscopic study. *Dysphagia.* 2014;29:199–203.
11. DePippo KL, Holas MA, Reding MJ. Validation of the 3-oz water swallow test for aspiration following stroke. *ArchNeurol.* 1992;49(12):1259–1261.
12. Daniels SK, Pathak S, Rosenbek JC, Morgan RO, Anderson JA. Rapid aspiration screening for suspected stroke: part 1: development and validation. *Arch Phys Med Rehabil.* 2016;97(9):1440–1448.
13. Edmiaston J, Connor LT, Steger-May K, Ford AL. A simple bedside stroke dysphagia screen, validated against videofluoroscopy, detects dysphagia and aspiration with high sensitivity. *J Stroke Cerebrovasc Dis.* 2014;23(4):712–716.
14. Wakasugi Y, Tohara H, Hattori F, et al. Screening test for silent aspiration at the bedside. *Dysphagia.* 2008;23(4):364–370.
15. Momosaki R, Abo M, Kakuda W, Kobayashi K. Applicability of the two-step thickened water test in patients with poststroke dysphagia: a novel assessment tool for paste food aspiration. *J Stroke Cerebrovasc Dis.* 2013;22(6):817–821.
16. Brodsky MB, Suiter DM, González-Fernández M, et al. Screening accuracy for aspiration using bedside water swallow tests: a systematic review and meta-analysis. *Chest.* 2016;150(1):148–163.
17. American Speech-Language-Hearing Association. Clinical indicators for instrumental assessment of dysphagia. 2000.
18. Stoschus B, Allescher HD. Drug-induced dysphagia. *Dysphagia.* 1993;8(2):154–159.
19. Al-Shehri AM. Drug-induced dysphagia. *Ann Saudi Med.* 2003;23(5):249–253.

20. Russell RI. Non-steroidal anti-inflammatory drugs and gastrointestinal damage —problems and solutions. *Postgrad Med J.* 2001;77(904):82–88.
21. Sebastian JL, McKinney WP, Kaufman J, Young MJ. Angiotensin-converting enzyme inhibitors and cough: prevalence in an outpatient medical clinic population. *Chest.* 1991;99(1);36–39.
22. Madhavan A, Carnaby GD, Crary, MA. "Food Sticking in My Throat": videofluoroscopic evaluation of a common symptom. *Dysphagia.* 2015;30(3):343–348.
23. Daniels SK, Brailey K, Priestly DH, Herrington LR, Weisberg LA, Foundas AL. Aspiration in patients with acute stroke. *Arch Phys Med Rehabil.* 1998;79(1):14–19.
24. Horner J, Massey EW, Riski JE, Lathrop DL, Chase KN. Aspiration following stroke: clinical correlates and outcome. *Neurology.* 1988;38(9):1359–1362.
25. Malandraki GA, Hind JA, Gangnon R, Logemann JA, Robbins J. The utility of pitch elevation in the evaluation of oropharyngeal dysphagia: preliminary findings. *Am J Speech Lang Pathol.* 2011;20(4):262–268.
26. Smith Hammond CA, Goldstein LB, Horner RD, et al. Predicting aspiration in patients with ischemic stroke: comparison of clinical signs and aerodynamic measures of voluntary cough. *Chest.* 2009;135(3):769–777.
27. Hammond CS, Goldstein L, Zajac D, Gray L, Davenport P, Bolser D. Assessment of aspiration risk in stroke patients with quantification of voluntary cough. *Neurology.* 2001;56(4):502–506.
28. Pitts T, Bolser D, Rosenbek J, Troche M, Sapienza C. Voluntary cough production and swallow dysfunction in Parkinson's disease. *Dysphagia.* 2008;23(3):297–301.
29. Hegland KW, Okun MS, Troche MS. Sequential voluntary cough and aspiration or aspiration risk in Parkinson's disease. *Lung.* 2014;192(4):601–608.
30. Bianchi C, Baiardi P, Khirani S, Cantarella G. Cough peak flow as a predictor of pulmonary morbidity in patients with dysphagia. *Am J Phys Med Rehabil.* 2012;91(9):783–788.
31. Addington WR, Stephens RE, Gilliland K, Miller SP. Tartaric acid-induced cough and the superior laryngeal nerve evoked potential. *Am J Phys Med Rehabil.* 1998;77(6):523–526.
32. Addington WR, Stephens RE, Gilliland K, Rodriguez M. Assessing the laryngeal cough reflex and the risk of developing pneumonia after stroke. *Arch Phys Med Rehabil.* 1999;80(2):150–154.
33. Addington WR, Stephens RE, Gilliland KA. Assessing the laryngeal cough reflex and the risk of developing pneumonia after stroke: an interhospital comparison. *Stroke.* 1999;30(6):1203–1207.
34. Nieto L, de Diego A, Perpiñá M, et al. Cough reflex testing with inhaled capsaicin in the study of chronic cough. *Resp Med.* 2003;97(4):393–400.
35. Miles A, Zeng IS, McLauchlan H, Huckabee M-L. Cough reflex testing in dysphagia following stroke: a randomized controlled trial. *J Clin Med Res.* 2013;5(3):222.
36. McCullough GH, Rosenbek JC, Wertz RT, McCoy S, Mann G, McCullough K. Utility of clinical swallowing examination measures for detecting aspiration post-stroke. *J Speech Lang Hear Res.* 2005;48(6):1280–1293.
37. McCullough GH, Wertz RT, Rosenbek JC. Sensitivity and specificity of clinical/bedside examination signs for detecting aspiration in adults subsequent to stroke. *J Commun Disord.* 2001;34(1-2):55–72.
38. Groves-Wright KJ, Boyce S, Kelchner L. Perception of wet vocal quality in identifying penetration/aspiration during swallowing. *J Speech Lang Hear Res.* 2010;53(3):620–632.

39. Waito A, Bailey GL, Molfenter SM, Zoratto DC, Steele CM. Voice-quality abnormalities as a sign of dysphagia: validation against acoustic and videofluoroscopic data. *Dysphagia.* 2011;26(2):125–134.
40. Leder SB, Suiter DM, Green BG. Silent aspiration risk is volume-dependent. *Dysphagia.* 2011;26(3):304–309.
41. Brodsky MB, Gonzalez-Fernandez M, Michtalki H, Frymark T, Venediktov R, Schooling T. Screening accuracy for aspiration using bedside water swallow tests: a systematic review and meta-analysis. *Chest.* 2016;150(1):148–163.
42. Dantas RO, Cook IJ, Dodds WJ, Kern MK, Lang IM, Brasseur JG. Biomechanics of cricopharyngeal bars. *Gastroenterology.* 1990;99(5):1269–1274.
43. Lester S, Langmore SE, Lintzenich CR, et al. The effects of topical anesthetic on swallowing during nasoendoscopy. *Laryngoscope.* 2013;123(7):1704–1708.
44. O'Dea MB, Langmore SE, Krisciunas GP, et al. Effect of lidocaine on swallowing during FEES in patients with dysphagia. *Ann Otol Rhinol Laryngol.* 2015;124(7): 537–544.
45. Leder SB, Ross DA, Briskin KB, Sasaki CT. A prospective, double-blind, randomized study on the use of a topical anesthetic, vasoconstrictor, and placebo during transnasal flexible fiberoptic endoscopy. *J Speech Lang Hear Res.* 1997;40(6):1352–1357.
46. Murray J, Langmore SE, Ginsberg S, Dostie A. The significance of accumulated oropharyngeal secretions and swallowing frequency in predicting aspiration. *Dysphagia.* 1996;11(2):99–103.
47. Donzelli J, Brady S, Wesling M, Craney M. Predictive value of accumulated oropharyngeal secretions for aspiration during video nasal endoscopic evaluation of the swallow. *Ann Otol Rhinol Laryngol.* 2003;112(5):469–475.
48. Aviv JE, Martin JH, Debell M, Keen MS, Blitzer A. Air pulse quantification of supraglottic and pharyngeal sensation: a new technique. *Ann Otol Rhinol Laryngol.* 1993;102(10):777–780.
49. Aviv JE, Kim T, Thomson JE, Sunshine S, Kaplan S, Close LG. Fiberoptic endoscopic evaluation of swallowing with sensory testing (FEESST) in healthy controls. *Dysphagia.* 1998;13(2):87–92.
50. Aviv JE, Kaplan ST, Thomson JE, Spitzer J, Diamond B, Close LG. The safety of flexible endoscopic evaluation of swallowing with sensory testing (FEESST): an analysis of 500 consecutive evaluations. *Dysphagia.* 2000;15(1):39–44.
51. Kaneoka A, Krisciunas GP, Walsh K, Raade AS, Langmore SE. A comparison of 2 methods of endoscopic laryngeal sensory testing: a preliminary study. *Ann Otol Rhinol Laryngol.* 2015;124(3):187–193.
52. Langmore, SE. *Endoscopic Evaluation and Treatment of Swallowing Disorders.* New York, NY: Thieme; 2001.
53. Leder SB, Acton LM, Lisitano HL, Murray JT. Fiberoptic endoscopic evaluation of swallowing (FEES) with and without blue-dyed food. *Dysphagia.* 2005;20(2): 157–162.
54. Belafsky PC, Postma GN, Daniel E, Koufman JA. Transnasal esophagoscopy. *Otolaryngol Head Neck Surg.* 2001;125(6):588–589.
55. Postma GN, Cohen JT, Belafsky PC, et al. Transnasal esophagoscopy: revisited (over 700 consecutive cases). *Laryngoscope.* 2005;115(2):321–323.
56. Reavis KM, Morris CD, Gopal DV, Hunter JG, Jobe BA. Laryngopharyngeal reflux symptoms better predict the presence of esophageal adenocarcinoma than typical gastroesophageal reflux symptoms. *Ann Surg.* 2004;239(6):849–858.

57. Howell RJ, Pate MB, Ishman SL, et al. Prospective multi-institutional transnasal esophagoscopy: predictors of a change in management. *Laryngoscope.* 2016; 126(12):2667–2671.
58. Odze RD. Pathology of the gastroesophageal junction. *Semin Diagn Pathol.* 2005;*22*(4), 256–265.
59. Cameron AJ, Souto EO, Smyrk TC. Small adenocarcinomas of the esophagogastric junction: association with intestinal metaplasia and dysplasia. *Am J Gastroenterol.* 2002;97(6):1375–1380.
60. Hvid-Jensen F, Pedersen L, Drewes AM, Sørensen HT, Funch-Jensen P. Incidence of adenocarcinoma among patients with Barrett's esophagus. *N Engl J Med.* 2011;365(15):1375–1383.
61. Fox MR, Bredenoord AJ. Oesophageal high-resolution manometry: moving from research into clinical practice. *Gut.* 2008;57(3):405–423.
62. Kessing BF, Smout AJPM, Bredenoord AJ. Clinical applications of esophageal impedance monitoring and high-resolution manometry. *Curr Gastroenterol Rep.* 2012;14(3):197–205.
63. Bredenoord AJ, Smout AJPM. High-resolution manometry. *Dig Liver Dis.* 2008; 40(3):174–181.
64. Wirth D, Kern B, Guenin MO, et al. Outcome and quality of life after open surgery versus endoscopic stapler-assisted esophagodiverticulostomy for Zenker's diverticulum. *Dis Esophagus.* 2006;19(4):294–298.
65. Lin L, Lv L, Wang Y, Zha X, Tang F, Liu X. The clinical features of foreign body aspiration into the lower airway in geriatric patients. *Clin Interv Aging.* 2014;9:1613–1618.
66. Dabu J, Lindner M, Azzam M, et al. A case of chronic cough and pneumonia secondary to a foreign body. *Case Rep Med.* 2017;3092623.
67. Orizio P, Cinquini M, Minetti S, et al. Chronic cough and eosinophilic esophagitis: an uncommon association. *Case Rep Gastroenterol.* 2011;5(2):497–501.
68. Roy-Ghanta S, Larosa DF, Katzka DA. Atopic characteristics of adult patients with eosinophilic esophagitis. *Clin Gastroenterol Hepatol.* 2008;6(5):531–535.
69. Kelly KJ, Lazenby AJ, Rowe PC, Yardley JH, Perman JA, Sampson HA. Eosinophilic esophagitis attributed to gastroesophageal reflux: improvement with an amino acid–based formula. *Gastroenterol.* 1995;109(5):1503–1512.
70. Gorriz-Gil C, Villarreal IM, Alvarez-Montero O, Rodriguez-Valiente A, Magaz M, Garcia-Berrocal JR. Eosinophilic esophagitis: a relevant entity for the otolaryngologist. *Acta Otorrinolaringol Esp.* 2016;67(3):167–178.
71. Smith JA, Houghton LA. The oesophagus and cough: laryngo-pharyngeal reflux, microaspiration and vagal reflexes. *Cough.* 2013;9(1):12.
72. Amaris M, Dua KS, Naini SR, Samuel E, Shaker R. Characterization of the upper esophageal sphincter response during cough. *Chest,* 2012;142(5):1229–1236.
73. Pohl D, Tutuian R. Achalasia: an overview of diagnosis and treatment. *Gastrointestin Liver Dis.* 2007;16(3):297–303.
74. Sinan H, Tatum RP, Soares RV, Martin AV, Pellegrini, CA, Oelschlager BK. Prevalence of respiratory symptoms in patients with achalasia. *Dis Esophagus.* 2011;24(4):224–228.
75. Kwon HY, Lim JH, Shin YW, Kim C-W. A case of chronic cough caused by achalasia misconceived as gastroesophageal reflux disease. *Allergy Asthma Immunol Res.* 2014;6(6):573–576.

76. Gupta M, Ghoshal UC, Jindal S, Misra A, Nath A, Saraswat VA. Respiratory dysfunction is common in patients with achalasia and improves after pneumatic dilation. *Dig Dis Sci.* 2014;59(4):744–752.
77. Won HK, Yoon SJ, Song WJ. The double-sidedness of cough in the elderly. *Respir Physiol Neurobiol.* 2018;257:65–69
78. Morice AH, Jakes AD, Faruqi S, et al. A worldwide survey of chronic cough: a manifestation of enhanced somatosensory response. *Eur Respir J.* 2014;44(5): 1149–1155.
79. Dicpinigaitis PV. Clinical perspective—cough: an unmet need. *Curr Opin Pharmacol.* 2015;22:24–28.
80. Cook IJ. Oropharyngeal dysphagia. *Gastroenterol Clin North Am.* 2009;38(3): 411–431.
81. Humbert IA, Robbins J. Dysphagia in the elderly. *Phys Med Rehabil Clin North Am.*, 2008;19(4):853–866.
82. Andrews JM, Heddle R, Hebbard GS, Checklin H, Besanko L, Fraser RJ. Age and gender affect likely manometric diagnosis: audit of a tertiary referral hospital clinical esophageal manometry service. *J Gastroenterol Hepatol.* 2009; 24(1):125–128.
83. Gutschow CA, Leers JM, Schröder W, et al. Effect of aging on esophageal motility in patients with and without GERD. *Ger Med Sci.* 2011;9:Doc22.
84. Grande L, Lacima G, Ros E, et al. Deterioration of esophageal motility with age: a manometric study of 79 healthy subjects. *Am J Gastroenterol.* 1999;94(7): 1795–1801.
85. Gregersen H, Pedersen J, Drewes AM. Deterioration of muscle function in the human esophagus with age. *Dig Dis Sci.* 2008;53(12):3065–3070.
86. Ren J, Shaker R, Kusano M, et al. Effect of aging on the secondary esophageal peristalsis: presbyesophagus revisited. *Am J Physiol Gastrointest Liver Physiol.* 1995;268(5):G772–G779.
87. Besanko LK, Burgstad CM, Cock C, Heddle R, Fraser A, Fraser RJL. Changes in esophageal and lower esophageal sphincter motility with healthy aging. *J Gastrointestin Liver Dis.* 2014;23(3):243–248.
88. Allen J, White CJ, Leonard R, Belafsky PC. Effect of cricopharyngeus muscle surgery on the pharynx. *Laryngoscope.* 2010;120(8):1498–1503.
89. Sallam H, McNearney TA, Chen JD. Systematic review: pathophysiology and management of gastrointestinal dysmotility in systemic sclerosis (scleroderma). *Aliment Pharmacol Ther.* 2006:23(6);691–712.
90. Lim KG. Scleroderma lung-associated cough. *Chest.* 2012;142(3):556–557.
91. Sloan JA, Mulki R, Sandhu N, Samuel S, Katz PO. Jackhammer esophagus: symptom presentation, associated distal contractile integral, and assessment of bolus transit. *J Clin Gastroenterol*. Published online March 7, 2018.
92. O'Rourke A, Humphries K. The use of high-resolution pharyngeal manometry as biofeedback in dysphagia therapy. *Ear Nose Throat J.* 2017;96(2):56–58.

8

COUGH MANAGEMENT: THE SPEECH-LANGUAGE PATHOLOGIST'S ROLE IN THE TREATMENT OF CHRONIC COUGH

Hadas Golan and Chandler C. Thompson

INTRODUCTION

A cough persisting for longer than 8 weeks, despite extensive medical investigation and treatment, is considered a chronic cough. Laryngeal dysfunction and laryngeal irritation are increasingly recognized in chronic persistent cough, with patients describing cough triggers related to phonation, swallowing, and/or respiration. Other laryngeal symptoms such as hoarseness, dyspnea, stridor, and globus commonly coexist with the cough.[1] There is evidence supporting the benefit of coordinated care between otolaryngology and speech-language pathology (SLP) in treating patients with chronic cough,[2,3] as symptoms are usually localized to the larynx.

Patients routinely report having consulted multiple specialists seeking information about causes and cures: primary care physicians, pediatricians, otolaryngologists, pulmonologists, allergists, gastroenterologists and psychologists. Working together with some or all of these physician collaborators, speech-language pathologists (SLPs) are uniquely trained and qualified to behaviorally treat voice, swallowing, and motor speech disorders, which enables them to detect and address abnormalities in laryngeal and respiratory function.[4]

In the voice-clinic setting, the treatment of chronic cough has become a significant part of the SLP caseload, and SLP intervention provides options for patients who have either exhausted conventional management or who may require behavioral management in conjunction with medical therapies.

In this chapter the literature related to the behavioral management of chronic cough and associated laryngeal conditions by SLPs will be reviewed. The assessment process of the behavioral manifestations associated with patient complaints will be described, and treatment options starting with traditional SLP approaches and continuing with less traditional but increasingly more commonly used modalities will be discussed.

Data from systematic review of nonpharmacological interventions for chronic cough by Chamberlain et al support the use of two to four speech therapy sessions that include education, cough suppression techniques, breathing exercises, vocal hygiene and hydration, and counseling. These interventions have been found to significantly reduce cough reflex sensitivity, in turn leading to reductions in cough severity and frequency, and improving the cough-related quality of life in people with chronic cough.[5] One randomized-control trial involving 87 patients with chronic cough demonstrated significant improvements in cough-symptom scores yielded by these interventions relative to control patients, who received healthy lifestyle advice and education alone.[6]

UNDERLYING MECHANISMS OF COUGH ADDRESSED IN SLP TREATMENT

SLP management of chronic cough is designed to increase patient self-efficacy in their ability to break the vicious cycle of cough-induced irritation. Lee et al describe cough as a "complex respiratory response," involving a mixture of involuntary brainstem reflexes and voluntary cortical control.[7] Studies on capsaicin-induced cough, and cough associated with upper respiratory tract infection (URTI), have shown that cough is under the control of the cerebral cortex and can be voluntarily inhibited or initiated.[8] Deliberate cough in response to laryngeal irritation, rather than for the purpose of clearing the lungs, may lead to a positive feedback loop in which irritation leads to coughing, causing more irritation, and so on, hypersensitizing the afferent nerve receptors that results in a decreased cough threshold. Speech pathology treatment aims to increase voluntary control of the cough and to reduce cough-reflex sensitivity.[1] Using capsaicin cough-sensitivity testing, ambulatory cough monitoring, and self-ratings of cough, Ryan et al demonstrated that the active suppression of cough raises the cough threshold. As their patients learned to voluntarily suppress their cough through speech pathology training and broke this cycle, their cough-reflex sensitivity and cough frequency lessened and their cough-related quality of life improved.[9]

UPPER AIRWAYS DISORDERS LINKED TO CHRONIC COUGH

Other laryngeal disorders often coexist in patients with chronic cough that affect their breathing, swallowing, and voice. There is a complex relationship among chronic cough, paradoxical vocal fold motion disorder (PVFMD) (also known as vocal cord dysfunction), globus pharyngeus, and muscle tension dysphonia (MTD). These conditions are, in part or in total, all viewed as manifestations of laryngeal hypersensitivity syndrome and respond similarly to speech pathology intervention.[1,10]

Several theoretical models have been proposed to better characterize these conditions. The irritable larynx syndrome (ILS) model, introduced by Morrison and Rammage,[11] proposes that ILS is a central sensitivity syndrome resulting from central neural plasticity due to nerve or tissue injury. This manifests as a normally structured larynx that is dysfunctional due to abnormal laryngeal posturing and palpable muscle tension involving intrinsic and extrinsic laryngeal muscles. Causes may include habitual muscle misuse, emotional distress, viral illness, and chronic gastroesophageal reflux (GER) stimulation. ILS occurs when the neuronal networks in the brainstem responsible for laryngeal control are maintained in a hyperexcitable state, resulting in an exaggerated response by the laryngeal and paralaryngeal muscles to normal sensory input. Associated symptoms can include episodic laryngospasm, MTD, globus pharyngeus, and chronic cough, and may be triggered by various stimuli. Murry et al proposed that chronic cough in patients with PVFMD was associated with aberrant laryngeal sensation; the larynx is actually edematous and desensitized from chronic acid irritation caused by LPR, leading to paradoxical adduction of the vocal folds during inspiration as a protective response against the inhalation of irritants.[12]

A second model, periodic occurrence of laryngeal obstruction (POLO), refers to episodic dyspnea as the primary symptom in response to triggers. In this model, cough is considered a concomitant symptom along with noisy breathing (stridor), chest and/or throat tightness, and dysphonia.[13] In a recently published article, Shembel et al proposed an integrated theoretical algorithmic paradigm classifying the key clinical features of this spectrum of disorders, termed episodic laryngeal breathing disorders (ELBDs). It includes clinical subgroups to explain the considerable individual variability in symptom presentations, laryngoscopic findings, and triggers. They called for an interdisciplinary approach to improve diagnostic criteria and for future study of the underlying pathophysiological mechanisms of ELBDs.[14]

Chronic cough has been associated with PVFMD. These two conditions may commonly co-occur: Chronic cough has been described in as many as 80% of patients with PVFMD.[15] In one study, patients with PVFMD had cough as the primary symptom in 59% of the subjects,[16] and in another, adduction of the vocal folds during inspiration was present in 56% of subjects with chronic cough.[17] Vertigan et al proposed a model depicting chronic cough and PVFMD on a continuum, with pure cough and pure PVFMD at either end of the continuum, and some combination of the two in the middle.[18] For this reason PVFMD will be included in the discussion of the evaluation and of the different treatment modalities of chronic cough later on in this chapter.

Once a patient has been appropriately referred to an SLP, a comprehensive evaluation will be conducted, leading to treatment recommendations.

EVALUATION

SLPs can play an important role in evaluating chronic cough, even if the etiology is unknown or multifactorial. In their book *Speech Pathology Management of Chronic Refractory Cough and Related Disorders,* Vertigan and Gibson describe inclusion and exclusion criteria for referral to an SLP for treatment of chronic cough and PVFMD.[1] These may be useful for healthcare providers to familiarize themselves with prior to making such a referral, especially so they are able to rule out serious underlying disease and/or to adjust the dosing of medication for asthma and GER, to substitute other medications for those that may themselves trigger cough (such as ACE inhibitors), and to consider testing for nonacid pepsin-induced pharyngeal reflux.

Inclusion criteria:

- Cough qualifies as chronic cough (8+ weeks since onset)
- Cough is problematic for the patient
- Cough persists despite medical treatment for common causes of cough

Exclusion criteria:

- Untreated asthma, GERD/LPR, allergies, rhinitis (can occur concurrently with SLP treatment)
- Current upper respiratory tract infection
- Spirometry not conducted; asthma not reviewed in last 2 years
- Trial of ACE inhibitor withdrawal not yet undertaken

- Patient not reviewed by/referred by respiratory physician or otolaryngologist

The American Speech-Language Hearing Association has provided an expertly vetted, consensus-based template for SLPs to use when assessing voice and laryngeal disorders. The questions included can help guide the practitioner in determining the overall function of the larynx.[19]

Case History

Information provided by the patient at the time of initial evaluation should include medical diagnosis, date of onset of cough, relevant medical and surgical history, medications, and allergies. Questionnaires such as the Cough Severity Index (CSI)[20] (Table 8–1), Leicester Cough Questionnaire (LCQ),[21] Voice Handicap Index-10 (VHI-10)[22] (Table 8–2), Dyspnea Index (DI)[23] (Table 8–3), and Reflux Symptom Index (RSI)[24] (Table 8–4) provide indications of the severity of the chronic cough and its impact on the patient's life.

Vocal hygiene information, including water, caffeine, alcohol and other beverage intake; smoking and recreational drug history; and vocal activities at work, at home, and socially, provide details that may help the SLP understand the patient's total laryngeal demand. Reflux history and exposure to environmental triggers (temperature changes, smoke, chemicals, and allergens) may also contribute valuable information.

In addition to questions about voice use, the clinician should also include questions about breathing and swallowing, as well as cough-specific questions such as:

- When did the cough start and was there any specific event associated with it?
- What happens just before you cough?
- Do you initiate the cough in response to irritation, or does the cough just "explode"?
- Are there specific events, settings, or severity of stress that usually trigger a coughing episode?
- What strategies have you used to try to suppress the cough, or to break a cycle of coughing?
- Has the severity and/or duration of a coughing episode caused urinary incontinence or vomiting?
- Is your cough triggered by talking, laughing, walking, or yawning?

Table 8–1. Cough Severity Index (CSI)

The Cough Severity Index (CSI) is a self-administered, 10-item outcomes instrument to quantify a patient's symptoms of chronic cough of upper airway origin. The total score ranges from 0 to 40 based on the sum of responses to 10 questions on a 5-point scale ranging from "never a problem" to "always a problem." A score of 3 or below is considered normal. A score higher than 3 means that the cough may be impacting quality of life.

	Never	Almost Never	Sometimes	Almost Always	Always
My cough is worse when I lie down.	0	1	2	3	4
My coughing problem causes me to restrict my personal and social life.	0	1	2	3	4
I tend to avoid places because of my coughing problem.	0	1	2	3	4
I feel embarrassed because of my coughing problem.	0	1	2	3	4
People ask, "What's wrong?" because I cough a lot.	0	1	2	3	4
I run out of air when I cough.	0	1	2	3	4
My coughing problem affects my voice.	0	1	2	3	4
My coughing problem limits my physical activity.	0	1	2	3	4
My coughing problem upsets me.	0	1	2	3	4
People ask me if I'm sick because I cough a lot.	0	1	2	3	4

- Is your cough triggered by eating in general? Eating specific foods?
- Do you have any difficulty swallowing saliva, certain food consistencies, or liquids?
- Do you have any difficulty breathing? Is it harder to breathe in or to breathe out?

Table 8–2. The Voice Handicap Index 10-Item (VHI-10)

The Voice Handicap Index 10-Item (VHI-10) is a self-administered, 10-item outcomes instrument to quantify patients' perception of their voice handicap. The total score ranges from 0 to 40 based on the sum of responses to 10 questions on a 5-point scale ranging from "never a problem" to "always a problem." No Impact = 0%; Moderate Impact = 50%; Significant Impact = 100%.					
	Never	**Almost Never**	**Sometimes**	**Almost Always**	**Always**
1. My voice makes it difficult for people to hear me.	0	1	2	3	4
2. People have difficulty understanding me in a noisy room.	0	1	2	3	4
3. People ask, "What's wrong with your voice?"	0	1	2	3	4
4. I feel as though I have to strain to produce voice.	0	1	2	3	4
5. My voice difficulties restrict my personal and social life.	0	1	2	3	4
6. The clarity of my voice is unpredictable.	0	1	2	3	4
7. I feel left out of conversation because of my voice.	0	1	2	3	4
8. My voice problem causes me to lose income.	0	1	2	3	4
9. My voice problem upsets me.	0	1	2	3	4
10. My voice makes me feel handicapped.	0	1	2	3	4

Table 8–3. Dyspnea Index (DI)

The Dyspnea Index (DI) is a self-administered, 10-item outcomes instrument to quantify severity of symptoms in upper airway dyspnea. Preliminary data suggest that a score of <7 can be considered normal and >10 is suggestive of PVFM. A change score of 8 has been shown to be meaningful.					
	Never	**Almost Never**	**Sometimes**	**Almost Always**	**Always**
I have trouble getting air in.	0	1	2	3	4
I feel tightness in my throat when I am having my breathing problem.	0	1	2	3	4
It takes more effort to breathe than it used to.	0	1	2	3	4
Changes in weather affect my breathing problem.	0	1	2	3	4
My breathing gets worse with stress.	0	1	2	3	4
I make sound/noise breathing in.	0	1	2	3	4
I have to strain to breathe.	0	1	2	3	4
My shortness of breath gets worse with exercise or physical activity.	0	1	2	3	4
My breathing problem makes me feel stressed.	0	1	2	3	4
My breathing problem causes me to restrict my personal and social life.	0	1	2	3	4

Sources:

1. De Guzman V, Ballif CL, Maurer R, Hartnick CJ, Raol N. Validation of the Dyspnea Index in adolescents with exercise-induced paradoxical vocal fold motion. *JAMA Otolaryngol Head Neck Surg.* 2014; 140(9):823–828.
2. Shembel AC, Hartnick, C, Bunting G, et al. Perceptual clinical features in exercise-induced laryngeal obstruction (EILO): towards improving diagnostic approaches. *Journal of Voice.* 2018.

Table 8–4. The RSI

The Reflux Symptom Index (RSI) is a self-administered, 9-item outcomes instrument to quantify symptoms in patients with laryngopharyngeal reflux (LPR). An RSI score of ≤13 can be considered normal. Some degree of reflux is present in normal individuals. A score >13 is suggestive of significant LPR symptoms.

	No Problem (0)	(1)	(2)	(3)	(4)	Severe Problem (5)
1. Hoarseness or a problem with your voice	0	1	2	3	4	5
2. Clearing your throat	0	1	2	3	4	5
3. Excess throat mucus or post nasal drip	0	1	2	3	4	5
4. Difficulty swallowing food, liquids, or pills	0	1	2	3	4	5
5. Coughing after you ate or while lying down	0	1	2	3	4	5
6. Breathing difficulties or choking episodes	0	1	2	3	4	5
7. Troublesome or annoying cough	0	1	2	3	4	5
8. Sensation of something sticking in your throat or a lump in your throat	0	1	2	3	4	5
9. Heartburn, chest pain, indigestion, or stomach acid coming up	0	1	2	3	4	5

SLP Clinician Observations

The evaluating clinician includes observations of posture, respiratory, cough-related and vocal behaviors. For example: Does the patient exhibit noisy breathing? Does talking trigger cough? Additional observations that may help the clinician structure the treatment plan include:

Breathing Pattern

- Diaphragmatic/upper chest/clavicular
- Inhalation:exhalation ratio
- Regular/irregular

- Route (mouth/nose)
- Breath holding
- Paradoxical abdominal movement during deep breathing
- Sighing, gasping, excessive yawning
- A lot of visible respiratory movement
- Breathing pattern change after a short exercise challenge
- Frequent throat clearing
- Speaking too long on one breath
- Running out of air when speaking

Voice-Use Habits

- Voice-use habits
- Loudness
- Rate of speech
- Pitch
- Resonance pattern

Muscle tension assessment noted by the SLP in the upper body, abdomen, neck, jaw, face, lips, or base of tongue may help to better understand patterns of dysfunction. This may be expanded to observation of the posture while seated and standing (addressed in detail later in this chapter), and observations made during laryngeal palpation, such as tenderness/pain, reduction in thyrohyoid space, elevation during speech, and whether or not laryngeal palpation elicits coughing.

Functional Measurements

Because dysphonia is common in chronic cough, voice assessment is part of the evaluation session. A comprehensive assessment including instrumental measures is indicated in individuals who report voice changes or present with dysphonia. For those with access to specialized equipment, analysis of acoustic and aerodynamic measures of laryngeal function can provide the evaluating clinician with objective data gathered during a prescribed menu of tasks, such as vowel prolongation, pitch glides, subglottal air pressure, mean airflow during voicing, and vital capacity, to name a few. These indirect measures of voice production offer a more complete understanding of laryngeal behavior and function and allow the clinician to make inferences about laryngeal and vocal fold physiology. In the hands of a skilled clinician with appropriate training and experience, these functional measures may also help determine etiology, diagnosis, severity, and measurable changes in vocal fold physiology after a course of therapy. [25]

Videostroboscopic evaluation of the larynx is done routinely in voice clinics to provide information regarding laryngeal structure and function. Laryngoscopy helps to detect abnormal laryngeal movements during respiration and phonation. The addition of a stroboscopic light source provides clinicians with the illusion of a slow-motion view of vocal fold vibration allowing them to detect subtle alterations in vibratory behavior of the vocal folds. Videostroboscopy is essential to rule out laryngeal pathology such as gross or subtle vocal fold lesions, mobility issues, or airway obstruction.[26] Laryngoscopy is also considered the gold standard for diagnosing PVFMD. If the patient is asymptomatic at the time of laryngoscopic examination, asking them to pant, breathe deeply, or to perform an exercise challenge, including something as sedentary as counting as quickly as possible from zero to 100 in as few breaths as possible, may sometimes elicit symptoms.[27]

Giliberto et al noted that in 80% of patients with chronic cough believed to be attributable to vagal neuropathy, vocal fold motion asymmetry was noted during videostroboscopic examination.[28]

For clinicians without a voice lab at their disposal, measures such as s:z ratio, maximum phonation time, presence of delayed onset, pitch glide, and average pitch during speech can offer insight into laryngeal behaviors. In addition, there are new smartphone applications and digital programs that can be downloaded and used by clinicians who invest the time to familiarize themselves with the technology.

TREATMENT

Traditional Speech Pathology Intervention

The rationale for speech therapy should be understood by the patient to increase motivation and compliance. Long-term goals of therapy are reducing laryngeal irritation affecting cough and improving voluntary control of cough and general control of respiratory symptoms,[6] so as to reduce and eliminate laryngeal and cough-reflex hypersensitivity,[1] and the frequency and severity of the cough. The SLP should also address posture and laryngeal, neck, and shoulder muscle tension.

Treatment paradigms for chronic cough described in the literature[2,3,6,10] employ techniques adapted from treating functional voice disorders and PVFMD, since the primary goals are similar for all three.

These may include:

- Patient education, identification of, and strategies to manage triggers of cough
- vocal hygiene
- cough suppression techniques
- postural modification
- respiratory retraining
- psychoeducational counseling
- voice therapy
- manual techniques to reduce paralaryngeal muscle tension.

Patient Education

Patients should be educated to recognize chronic cough as a manifestation of laryngeal hypersensitivity that doesn't serve any physiological function (ie, airway protection), and that continuous coughing lowers their cough threshold to such a level that coughing is triggered by progressively smaller stimuli. Learning that cough is both involuntary and voluntary helps to demystify the cough as a reflex beyond the patient's control and increases patient willingness to accept behavioral therapy.

Reviewing the patient's answers on the CSI (and VHI-10, DI, and RSI, where applicable) will give the SLP insight into the impact of cough and priorities for each individual patient, furthering the paradigm of treating the patient and not just the disorder. The patient and the SLP should work together to identify all of the steps involved in the pattern of chronic cough that has developed, and the SLP will teach strategies to break the cycle at any of the points identified.

Vocal Hygiene

Vocal hygiene counseling targets reduction of laryngeal irritation to minimize stimulation of cough receptors, and improvement of hydration. SLPs can provide dietary counseling, promote behavioral management of previously diagnosed acid reflux, encourage smoking cessation and the reduction of secondhand tobacco smoke exposure, and promote nasal breathing to reduce laryngeal dryness and irritation. Helping a patient to identify vocal behaviors that may trigger a cough, such as speaking too long on one breath, or speaking at a consistently loud volume, may reduce the demands made on the larynx and contribute to decreasing the frequency and duration of the cough.

SLPs in the clinical setting often describe systemic and surface hydration as beneficial for vocal fold health. Most SLPs include recommendations about optimal hydration (64 ounces of water intake daily), avoiding presumed drying substances such as caffeine (not supported in the literature), and use of humidified air to improve vocal function. However, there is no conclusive evidence this is true, and more targeted research is needed to study the biological mechanisms influencing vocal fold hydration before a conclusive hydration regimen can be validated.[29]

A literature review across many disciplines by Hartley and Thibeault revealed that there is no clear understanding of the underlying mechanisms regarding the effects of euhydration (normal state of body water content/absence of relative hydration or dehydration), hypohydration, or hyperhydration across the lifespan, or of the connection between surface and systemic hydration.[29] However, literature about vocal health has successfully demonstrated, in both animal and human-subject studies, the ill effects of both surface and systemic dehydration, primarily related to increased effort of phonation. Clinical advice regarding adequate surface hydration for patients with chronic cough may be based on studies showing that known cough behaviors, such as rapid deep breathing through the mouth or the breathing of poorly humidified air, can lead to dehydration of tissues in the larynx, increasing laryngeal dryness and irritation and vocal effort.[30]

Strategies to Control the Cough

SLPs use various breathing retraining programs and cough suppression techniques to address cough with or without PVFMD.

Cough Suppression or Distracting Techniques

With these techniques, patients learn to identify the physical sensations that precede the cough, such as a tickle, and try to suppress or delay the cough. They can implement one of the following symptom control techniques according to their preference:

- Substitute the throat clear or cough with an effortful swallow (dry or with water), swallow while manually lowering the larynx, sucking on ice, or sucking a nonmedicated, sugar-free lozenge to increase the frequency of saliva swallows, in an attempt to delay the cough.
- Sniff to inhale and abduct the vocal folds (some suggest a brisk sniff, others recommend a slow, drawn-out inhalation).

- Pursed lip breathing (PLB): exhale through pursed lips or gentle prolonged fricatives in order to maximize expiratory flow through the larynx and provide positive-end expiratory pressure to maintain the vocal folds in an abducted/separated position.
- Inhaling with PLB or through a straw helps to regulate the airflow and shift the constriction to the lips rather than the larynx.[31]

Laryngeal Deconstriction Techniques

- "Silent laughing" adapted from the Estill Voice Model. With this, patients increase their awareness of laryngeal constriction by contrasting it with an open-throat sensation and learn how to maintain the open throat posture. This may also help to improve awareness of breath holding patterns, which themselves may trigger cough or PVFM episode.[32]
- Relaxed throat breathing designed to shift attention away from the larynx by emphasizing diaphragmatic breathing, and to maintain vocal fold abduction throughout the breathing cycle to prevent adduction and consequent cough. Patients are guided to release tension in the upper body, shoulders, neck, jaw, and abdominal muscles, maintain an open throat sensation, and notice the gentle natural expansion and deflation in the diaphragm and or abdominal area.[33]

Patients are instructed to practice these techniques frequently during their daily activities when asymptomatic to facilitate automatic recall at the first sense of the urge to cough. Lastly, they are gradually exposed to their known triggers in the clinic in order to desensitize the cough response.[1]

Posture

Postural alignment is an important component in treating and optimizing respiratory and laryngeal function.[34] Respiratory muscles have a dual function in both posture and spinal stabilization, and there are close links between breathing and musculoskeletal function. Habitually poor posture such as a slumping over may compromise the action of the diaphragm by abdominal compression.[35] Alternately, posture may be influenced by altered breathing patterns. Solow et al. noted that children who are mouth breathers due to obstructed upper airways, for example, commonly exhibit habitual forward head posture (FHP) to increase the size of the airways and to facilitate breathing.[36–38] Moreover, FHP is known to influence respiratory function by weakening respiratory muscles such as the sternocleidomastoid (SCM), scalene, and trapezius muscles, as well as increasing muscle tension around the thoracic spine and reducing its mobility. FHP and associated chronic neck pain have been shown in studies to reduce vital capacity.[39,40]

Regarding laryngeal function, postural imbalances in the neck and head structures can have a strong effect on vocal effort, and even subtle shifts in the position of the head may significantly impact the efficiency of laryngeal movement.[41] Patients with MTD often have excessive tension in their extrinsic or paralaryngeal musculature, which leads to the elevation of the larynx in the neck. Additionally, a disturbed alignment of the laryngeal cartilages (hyoid, thyroid, cricoid, and arytenoid) may affect the intrinsic laryngeal muscles, which in turn may alter the tension of the vocal folds, impairing control and resonance of the voice.[34,42] It is the authors' anecdotal clinical observation that patients with PVFM, chronic cough, and globus share similar dysfunctional postural and muscle patterns that may aggravate their laryngeal symptoms.

It is also observed that patients with a global postviral vagal neuropathy with chronic cough may also demonstrate a vocal fold paresis with MTD secondary to glottic insufficiency that ultimately leads to the changes previously mentioned; thus, it is not always clear if these changes are primary or secondary problems.[43]

SLPs should try to facilitate optimal postural alignment, which allows ease, freedom, and flexibility. They should also address the ergonomics of the patients' regular activities and encourage awareness of posture throughout the day. In more serious spinal conditions, a referral to a physical therapist is warranted.

Respiratory Retraining

Inspiratory muscle strength training devices (IMT) have been suggested for management of PVFMD and chronic cough.

Inspiratory muscle training has been shown to improve inspiratory muscle strength and to reduce the sensation of exertional dyspnea. IMT may facilitate a more desirable respiratory pattern and promote improved diaphragm relaxation and mechanical efficiency.[44] The use of IMT for people with chronic cough warrants further research.

Comprehensive breathing retraining programs, such as the Buteyko breathing technique, are described later in the chapter. Their goal is to restore physiologically normal minute and tidal volume and to correct carbon dioxide (CO_2) levels.

Psychoeducational Counseling

Motivational Interviewing (MI) is an evidence-based, person-centered counselling style used to increase intrinsic motivation by helping patients to explore and to resolve ambivalence to change.[45] SLPs can effectively use

MI techniques to increase patients' adherence to cough behavioral therapy and to facilitate behavioral changes.[46]

Instead of taking responsibility for changing patient behavior, the SLP uses MI techniques to support and empower the patient to take an active role in their healing process. Through thinking and talking about the patient's reasons for and means of making changes and supporting their self-efficacy—the belief they can achieve change—MI complements and ensures sustainability of treatment.

The SLP may address emotional issues associated with the cough and refer the patient to a mental health professional when these exceed the SLP's scope of practice.

Voice Therapy

Voice therapy can be effective for patients with chronic cough in the following ways:

- Cough and throat clearing are considered phonotraumatic behaviors that may cause vocal fold edema or hemorrhage, or lesions such as nodules and polyps. Clinically significant voice disorders are present in up to 40% of patients with chronic cough and PVFMD.[1]
- The movement of the vocal folds or an alteration in the normal movement with glottic insufficiency [47]and a patient's pattern of phonation, such as hyperadduction, may stimulate pressure receptors in the larynx enough to trigger cough.[1]
- Inflammatory mediators have been shown to increase following vocally fatiguing tasks and to decrease following resonant voice therapy, indicating that airway inflammation can be affected negatively or positively by phonatory patterns, therefore affecting cough.[1]
- Supraglottic constriction, which is present in primary MTD and is more likely evidence of secondary MTD due to glottic insufficiency, might sometimes act as an irritant and result in throat clearing or cough. MTD often makes it feel as if there is something in the throat, especially when swallowing. The concept of muscle tension dysphagia is novel but requires further research and understanding but may be a significant contributor to the globus sensation.[48]
- Cough often subsides when MTD is resolved.[1]

Voice symptoms may themselves resolve following treatment of the cough if they were integral to the cough. If not, dysphonia is likely a separate condition and needs to be treated.[1]

NEW MODALITIES IN THE TREATMENT OF COUGH

SLPs often consider the use of expanded modality therapies beyond those taught in SLP graduate programs, such as hypnosis, manual techniques, and Buteyko breathing techniques. The three modalities we have chosen to highlight below require special training.

Hypnosis

Hypnosis has been shown as a viable tool in the treatment of chronic cough. Defined as "a state of consciousness involving focused attention and reduced peripheral awareness characterized by an enhanced capacity for response to suggestion,"[49] hypnosis has been officially recognized by the American Medical Association as a legitimate medical tool since 1958. This shift in consciousness enables the person to tap into the natural abilities and allows them to more easily modify sensations, perceptions, thoughts, feelings, and behaviors.

A hypnotic state is usually established by an induction procedure. Most inductions include suggestions for relaxation, calmness, and well-being. People experience hypnosis differently, with some describing it as an altered state of consciousness, and others as a relaxed state of focused attention resembling a meditative state.[50] Contrary to common myths and misconceptions regarding hypnosis, people who have been hypnotized do not lose control over their behavior, and usually remember what transpired during hypnosis.

The American Society of Clinical Hypnosis (ASCH) offers certification programs for licensed practitioners, including SLPs.

A retrospective chart review described 56 children and adolescents with habit cough who were treated in two different institutions by a pediatric pulmonologist or a child psychologist. In 78% of these patients, the cough resolved during or immediately after the initial hypnosis session, and within a month, an additional 12% of the patients experienced resolution of their cough. The patients were followed for an average of 13 months. The cough recurred 1 to 3 times in 22% of the patients, and all but one used hypnosis to manage it. The authors concluded that self-hypnosis offers a safe, efficient means of resolving habit cough.[51]

Manual Techniques

Elevated laryngeal position in the pharynx has repeatedly been noted to contribute to or, possibly more accurately stated, is one of the physical representations of MTD. This is why traditional voice therapy includes manual circumlaryngeal techniques intended to reduce musculoskeletal tension and hyperfunction by re-posturing the larynx.[52,53] This treatment involves kneading the extralaryngeal musculature in an anterior-posterior direction at specific locations while exerting a downward pull on the larynx while the patient is phonating.

Behavioral therapy incorporating manual laryngeal reposturing by an experienced voice clinician has been shown to be an effective primary modality for MTD with consistently improved perceptual and acoustic measurements of vocal function during the follow-up period.[54] Anecdotally, people with chronic cough often report that the lower laryngeal position following these techniques allows for a stronger swallow, which helps them to clear mucus more effectively and reduce laryngeal irritation.

More recently, some specialized SLPs have been utilizing holistic and comprehensive physical therapy and osteopathic manual therapy techniques such as myofascial release (MFR) to facilitate improved respiratory and laryngeal function. Osteopathic principles and practice are based upon the interrelationship of structure and function and the body's natural ability to self-regulate and heal itself.[37,55] There are different ideas about how manual therapy works, and researchers and clinicians are now beginning to look at issues of swallow and voice from a more neurocentric perspective. Tight muscles are the result of protective responses produced by the nervous system. Manual therapists use the skin and deeper structures to affect neural tension via accepted neurodynamic techniques.

When clinicians apply manual therapy/MFR to a patient with issues of chronic cough, they may be treating neuromuscular tension generated as a result of injury, disuse, surgery, or chronic disease.[56] Additionally, this "safe touch" may reduce tension, allowing the muscles to relax and to communicate this relaxed state to the nervous system. When the nervous system no longer receives the feedback loop indicating a need for "protection," it can instruct the muscle tone to change from hypertonic to a more normal tone.[57]

To further address excessive overall body tension, SLPs may encourage patients to become more aware of their specific tension-holding patterns, and to monitor these throughout the day. Patients can learn different strategies to release neck, tongue, and jaw tension, such as stretches and self-circumlaryngeal massage.

Dysfunctional Breathing and the Buteyko Breathing Method

This section will outline dysfunctional breathing (DB), discuss its parameters and its symptoms, and show the connection between DB and chronic cough/PVFMD. It will also describe how correcting DB can help with chronic cough/PVFMD, and introduce the Buteyko method as a means for addressing DB.

Chronic cough and other laryngeal conditions such as PVFMD and globus have been linked to DB and are among the most common symptoms associated with it.[58] There is no consensus on a precise definition of DB, but the term generally describes breathing disorders where chronic or recurrent changes in breathing pattern cause respiratory and nonrespiratory symptoms in absence or in excess of organic respiratory or cardiac disease.[59,60] The disordered breathing pattern may reflect abnormalities in rate or depth of breathing, or in breathing mechanics that may involve the nose, oropharynx, larynx, chest wall muscles, and/or diaphragm.[60] PVFMD is considered a form of DB.[61] Barker and Everard proposed that DB can be subdivided into either thoracic or extrathoracic forms. Thoracic DB is characterized by predominantly upper chest breathing. Extrathoracic DB involves the upper airway in addition to the upper thoracic breathing pattern, and includes PVFMD and exercise-induced laryngomalacia.[61] Dysfunctional breathing may contribute to disproportionate dyspnea and other medically "unexplained" symptoms that don't respond to asthma medications.[62]

Some of the older literature focused on hyperventilation syndrome (HVS) and hypocapnia; however, it is recognized now that HVS and its associated signs and symptoms cannot always be attributed to, and have weak correlations with, CO_2 levels. Instead, a broader characterization of symptoms should include the biochemical, biomechanical, and psychophysiological dimensions of breathing.[63] The biochemical dimension refers to hyperventilation with symptoms arising from respiratory alkalosis and hypocapnia. The biomechanical dimension refers to respiratory muscle and breathing pattern dysfunction, and the psychophysiological dimension refers to interactions of physiology with mental and emotional factors. These dimensions can be related or distinct and produce the unexplained symptoms.[64]

Symptoms of Dysfunctional Breathing

Dysfunctional breathing can affect individuals in different ways. Some people complain of mental distress; others may experience musculoskeletal and physical symptoms such as neck and shoulder problems, chronic pain, and fatigue. Many report a combination of both mental and physical factors.[65]

Biochemical changes in the body due to DB may seriously impact emotional well-being, circulation, digestive function, and the musculoskeletal structures involved in respiration.[37] DB may result in: cough, significant dyspnea, chest pain and tightness, exercise-induced breathlessness, frequent yawning or sighing, anxiety, lightheadedness, palpitations, muscle spasm, and fatigue.

Nonrespiratory neurovascular symptoms such as dizziness, numbness and tingling have the strongest relationship to low CO_2, the biochemical dimension of breathing.

Respiratory symptoms such as inability to take a deep breath, chest tightness, and shortness of breath are typically related to the biomechanical and psychophysiological dimensions of DB.[64]

Prevalence of Dysfunctional Breathing

It has been estimated that DB affects approximately 5% to 11% of the general population,[37,66] 20% to 64% of adults with asthma,[61,64,66,67] and up to 83% of people with anxiety.[68]

DB often coexists with and exacerbates symptoms of asthma,[61,66,67,69] chronic obstructive pulmonary disease (COPD), rhinosinusitis, pain, cardiovascular disease, headaches, and migraines.[37]

Diagnosis of Dysfunctional Breathing

The diagnosis of DB first requires the exclusion and/or treatment of organic pathology. Only then can a functional diagnosis be entertained.[70] A variety of methods may be used to evaluate breathing function clinically, including instrumentation, observation, and palpation.

End-tidal capnography measures end-tidal carbon dioxide ($ETCO_2$) in exhaled nasal air to determine the presence of chronic or intermittent hyperventilation. $ETCO_2$ correlates with alveolar carbon dioxide concentration ($PACO_2$), which in turn correlates with arterial levels of CO_2 ($PaCO_2$). Capnography also provides information about respiratory rate and rhythm, and whether the breathing is smooth and rhythmical or choppy and irregular.[37,71]

Breath-holding time (BHT) at the end of a normal expiration is a measure of the dyspneic threshold. Low BHT is a common finding in people with DB.[59,72,73]

The Manual Assessment of Respiratory Motion (MARM) is a manual procedure used for assessing chest and abdominal movement during breathing. It quantifies the extent of thoracic breathing. The examiner can also gauge various aspects of breathing such as rate, volume, and regularity.[74]

Symptoms questionnaires such as the Nijmegen questionnaire (NQ)[63] and the Self-Evaluation of Breathing Questionnaire (SEBQ)[63] have been developed to evaluate all dimensions of breathing-related symptoms and their severity.

An accurate diagnosis in itself can provide significant reassurance and relief of anxiety, and may reduce symptoms.[59]

Hyperventilation and PVFM/Vocal Cord Dysfunction (VCD)

Hyperventilation is common among patients with PVFMD, and likely accounts for symptoms of lightheadedness, visual changes, numbness, tingling, extremity heaviness, dizziness, and near-syncope or syncope described by these patients. The $PaCO_2$ of patients with PVFMD is typically lower than normal because of the hyperventilation that accompanies most attacks.[75] In a retrospective study of 54 patients with exercise-induced PVFMD, 76% had concomitant hyperventilation as measured by a symptom questionnaire. An end-tidal CO_2 of less than 30 mm Hg, a physiologic consequence of hyperventilation, was seen in 48% of the patients.[76]

It is interesting to note that clinics use voluntary hyperventilation when trying to provoke PVFM symptoms during the laryngeal exam. The fact that cough and PVFM symptoms can be reproduced by hyperventilation suggests that hyperventilation may contribute to symptoms. Parker and

Berg have suggested that hyperventilation may be a possible mechanism for explaining PVFMD and may require alternative therapeutic approaches in people unresponsive to traditional SLP therapy.[76] The Buteyko breathing program discussed next is designed to reverse hyperventilation and may be a viable treatment option for these patients.

Buteyko Breathing Retraining

Breathing retraining taught primarily by specialized physical therapists and SLP is recognized as the first line of treatment for patients with DB.[77,61]

One form of respiratory retraining is the Buteyko Breathing Technique (BBT). It is based on Ukranian physician Dr. Konstantin Buteyko's theories that many symptoms and disease processes may be caused by chronic "overbreathing" or hidden hyperventilation, and the resultant CO_2 deficiency. Due to the Bohr effect, the lowered levels of CO_2 inhibit the release of oxygen from hemoglobin to the tissue cells which, in turn, may lead to ischemia, fatigue, and other symptoms.[78] BBT is an educational program designed to restore normal breathing patterns. It consists of breathing exercises and lifestyle factors of physical exercise, food, speech, and sleeping as they relate to healthy breathing.

The BBT's approach for cough management is similar to the traditional SLP management of cough suppression and restoring relaxed nasal diaphragmatic breathing. In the context of the BBT theoretical model, cough can manifest as both the cause and effect of overbreathing. The BBT intends to address the underlying causes of overbreathing, while SLP intervention for cough is designed to addresses symptoms.[6]

The BBT aims to reprogram the respiratory center to adapt to higher levels of CO_2 and thus to improve the symptoms caused by the chronic hyperventilation. BBT exercises involve the voluntary reduction of the volume of breathing through the relaxation of the respiratory muscles in combination with breath-holding techniques. The improvement in breathing control and function experienced with the BBT may be explained by mechanisms other than raising CO_2 alone. For example, the biomechanical problem of hyperinflation of the lungs and the anxiety surrounding symptoms are both likely to decrease with this treatment methodology.[64]

The BBT is best known as a treatment for asthma. Several clinical trials on BBT showed that patients substantially reduced their medication use with no deterioration in lung function and improvement in asthma symptoms.[79–81] The BBT is also used as a supportive therapy for people with chronic mouth breathing, nasal symptoms, COPD, obstructive sleep apnea and snoring, and stress-related disorders. Its principles and techniques are also increasingly being used to help improve athletic performance.[82]

To address chronic cough, patients are educated about the negative impact that excessive breathing and harsh cough can have on the tissue linings of the nose, throat, and lungs. These can cause dehydration and inflammation of the tissues and, consequently, an increase in mucus production to protect the drying airways. With ongoing overbreathing, this mucus may thicken and become harder to clear, exacerbating the original cough, creating a vicious cycle (Figure 8–1). Mouth breathing, common in patients with chronic cough,[3] may also cause the throat to become dry and raw if sustained, causing a tickling sensation, which patients report often leads to coughing. This can cause a persistent cycle of dry throat, coughing, irritated and dry throat, coughing, and so on. Coughing is considered a hyperventilation behavior because of the excessive loss of CO_2 with the fast and forceful exhalation followed by the large inhalation through the mouth, often repeatedly as in coughing fits. The excessive loss of CO_2 aggravates smooth muscle constriction in the airways of susceptible people.[37,83]

The BBT emphasizes establishing and maintaining gentle nasal breathing at all times, including during exercise, speech inhalation, and sleep. This may be beneficial for patients with chronic cough, since studies have shown that as many as 50% of these patients are habitual mouth breathers, which may, in turn, further exacerbate laryngeal symptoms.[3,84] As gentle nasal breathing is habituated, tissue dryness and irritation and excessive mucus production may diminish, allowing the cough to subside.

Nasal breathing may improve lung function and reduce asthma exacerbations.[85] In one study of young people with asthma who were required to breathe only through the nose during exercise, post-exercise bronchoconstriction was almost completely inhibited. When instructed to breathe only through the mouth during exercise, an increased bronchoconstriction occurred, as measured by spirometry, flow-volume relationships, and body plethysmography.[86]

Open-mouth breathing caused by chronic nasal obstruction has also been identified as a risk factor for the collapse of the pharyngeal airway and may also be an important factor in the pathogenesis of obstructive sleep apnea. The airway dilator muscles lose some of their efficiency when the mouth is open. With nasal breathing, neural activity in the airway dilator muscles stabilizes the upper airway.[87] Future research is needed to explore how similar mechanisms may also affect the upper airways in PVFMD and cough.

Another way in which BBT reduces chronic cough is related to the psychological triggers, which may coexist and in many cases have been implicated in chronic cough.[1] Current research associates emotional disorders with decreased vagal tone as indicated by heart rate variability.[88] Breathing modification has been suggested to balance the autonomic nervous system by reducing sympathetic and increasing parasympathetic nervous system activity. This may assist with recovery and restoration of function in body systems disturbed by stress.[89]

Despite the relation of the BBT's core principles with its stated outcomes as proven by external studies, the BBT therapy itself has not been empirically tested for the treatment of chronic cough without asthma.

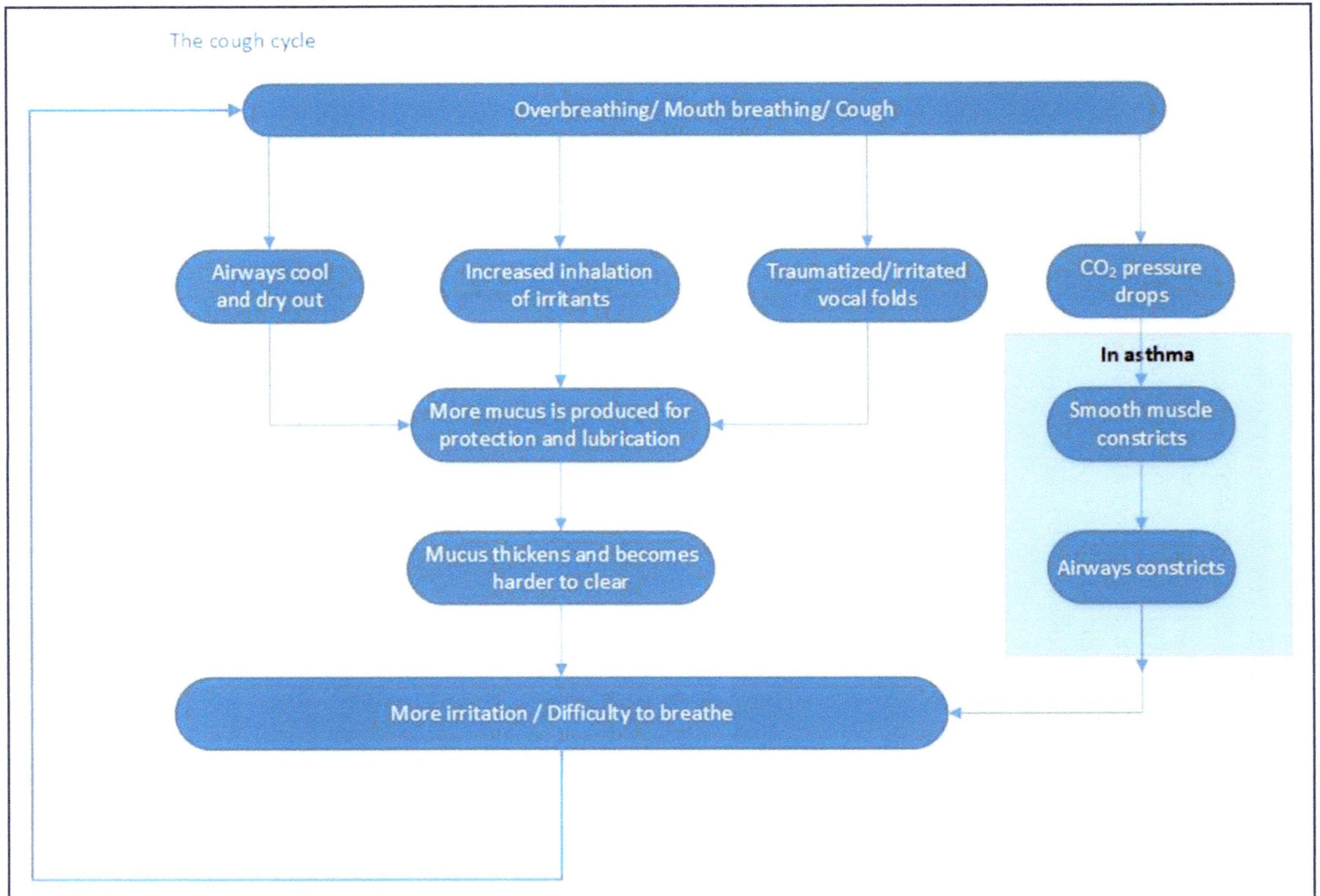

Figure 8–1. The Cough Cycle Chart.

CONCLUSION

The role of the SLP in the treatment of chronic cough is to reframe the patient's understanding of chronic cough and assist them in regaining laryngeal control. The SLP, working in conjunction with other multidisciplinary team members, will assess and treat the behavioral aspects associated with chronic cough, and may be able to improve the accuracy of diagnosis and the effectiveness of treatment.

THINKING OUTSIDE OF THE BOX

Medically unexplained dyspnea is commonly seen in outpatient clinics, and many physicians are uncomfortable managing these patients. When patients don't respond to the initial medical treatment, they often undergo extensive and unproductive investigations.[90]

Dysfunctional breathing, discussed in this chapter, should be considered as a causative or aggravating factor in these patients. The data about the prevalence of DB in people with respiratory disease presented in this review are likely low, mainly because their symptoms are usually attributed to their underlying disease, in turn resulting in an inappropriately high utilization of medications. In others, the symptoms are often attributed to anxiety and stress, with no consideration of the underlying biochemical and biomechanical influences.[61]

Considering the side effects, complications, and high costs of medical care, we propose a new clinical pathway involving SLPs to address DB and attempting to reestablish physiological balance. We propose that the treatment of DB be considered early in the management of the patient, especially in conditions for which breathing retraining has been proven effective, and/or when patients prefer natural therapies or behavioral management, or do not adhere to their medical treatment. Additional clinical research is needed to confirm this paradigm.

TAKE-HOME POINTS

- Medical evaluation and initiation of management of identifiable medical causes of chronic cough must occur prior to a referral to an SLP.
- Voice disorders and paradoxical vocal fold motion may co-occur with chronic cough, requiring a multipronged approach to treatment by the SLP.

- A comprehensive approach to treatment of chronic cough should incorporate traditional and nontraditional methods, including techniques utilized by SLPs.

REFERENCES

1. Vertigan A, Gibson PG. *Speech Pathology Management of Chronic Refractory Cough and Related Disorders*. Devon, UK: Compton Publishing; 2016.
2. Soni RS, Ebersole B, Jamal N. Treatment of chronic cough. *Otolaryngol Head Neck Surg*. 2017;156(1):103–108.
3. Murry T, Sapienza C. The role of voice therapy in the management of paradoxical vocal fold motion, chronic cough, and laryngospasm. *Otolaryngol Clin North Am*, 2010;43(1):73–83, viii-ix.
4. Petty BE, Dailey SH. The collaborative medical and behavioral management of chronic cough. *Perspect Voice Voice Dis*. 2009;19(2):49.
5. Chamberlain S, Birring SS, Garrod R. Nonpharmacological interventions for refractory chronic cough patients: systematic review. *Lung*. 2014;192(1):75–85.
6. Vertigan AE, Theodoros DG, Gibson PG, Winkworth AL. Efficacy of speech pathology management for chronic cough: a randomised placebo controlled trial of treatment efficacy. *Thorax*. 2006;61(12):1065–1069.
7. Lee PC, Cotterill-Jones C, Eccles R. Voluntary control of cough. *Pulm Pharmacol Ther*. 2002;15(3):317–320.
8. Hutchings HA, Eccles R, Smith AP, Jawad MS. Voluntary cough suppression as an indication of symptom severity in upper respiratory tract infections. *Eur Respir J*. 1993;6(10):1449–1454.
9. Ryan NM, Vertigan AE, Bone S, Gibson PG. Cough reflex sensitivity improves with speech-language pathology management of refractory chronic cough. *Cough*. 2010;6:5.
10. Gibson PG, Vertigan AE. Management of chronic refractory cough. *BMJ*. 2015;351:h5590.
11. Morrison M, Rammage L, Emami AJ. The irritable larynx syndrome. *J Voice*. 1999;13(3):447–455.
12. Murry T, Branski RC, Yu K, Cukier-Blaj S, Duflo S, Aviv JE. Laryngeal sensory deficits in patients with chronic cough and paradoxical vocal fold movement disorder. *Laryngoscope*. 2010;120(8):1576–1581.
13. Christopher KL, Morris MJ. Vocal cord dysfunction, paradoxic vocal fold motion, or laryngomalacia? Our understanding requires an interdisciplinary approach. *Otolaryngol Clin North Am*. 2010;43(1):43–66, viii.
14. Shembel AC, Sandage MJ, Verdolini Abbott K. Episodic laryngeal breathing disorders: literature review and proposal of preliminary theoretical framework. *J Voice*. 2017;31(1):125.e7–125.e16.
15. Murry T, Tabaee A, Aviv JE. Respiratory retraining of refractory cough and laryngopharyngeal reflux in patients with paradoxical vocal fold movement disorder. *Laryngoscope*. 2004;114(8):1341–1345.
16. Andrianopoulos MV, Gallivan GJ, Gallivan KH. PVCM, PVCD, EPL, and irritable larynx syndrome: what are we talking about and how do we treat it? *J Voice*. 2000;14(4):607–618.

17. Ryan NM, Gibson PG. Characterization of laryngeal dysfunction in chronic persistent cough. *Laryngoscope.* 2009;119(4):640–645.
18. Vertigan AE, Theodoros DG, Gibson PG, Winkworth AL. The relationship between chronic cough and paradoxical vocal fold movement: a review of the literature. *J Voice.* 2006;20(3):466–480.
19. Speech-Language-Hearing Association (ASHA). *Voice evaluation template.* https://www.asha.org/uploadedFiles/AATVoiceEvaluation.pdf. Published 2018. Accessed April 14, 2018.
20. Shembe, AC, Rosen CA, Zullo TG, Gartner-Schmidt JL. Development and validation of the Cough Severity Index: a severity index for chronic cough related to the upper airway. *Laryngoscope.* 2013;123(8):1931–1936.
21. Birring SS, Prudon B, Carr AJ, Singh SJ, Morgan MD, Pavord ID. Development of a symptom specific health status measure for patients with chronic cough: Leicester Cough Questionnaire (LCQ). *Thorax.* 2003;58(4):339–343.
22. Rosen CA, Lee AS, Osborne J, Zullo T, Murry T. Development and validation of the Voice Handicap Index-10. *Laryngoscope.* 2004;114(9):1549–1556.
23. Gartner-Schmidt JL, Shembel AC, Zullo TG, Rosen CA. Development and validation of the Dyspnea Index (DI): a severity index for upper airway-related dyspnea. *J Voice.* 2014;28(6):775–782.
24. Belafsky PC, Postma GN, Koufman JA. Validity and reliability of the Reflux Symptom Index (RSI). *J Voice.* 2002;16(2):274–277.
25. Stemple JC, Roy N, Klaben B. *Clinical Voice Pathology: Theory and Management.* San Diego, CA: Plural Publishing; 2014.
26. Bless DM, Hirano M, Feder RJ. Videostroboscopic evaluation of the larynx. *Ear Nose Throat J.* 1987;66(7):289–296.
27. Koufman JA, Block C. Differential diagnosis of paradoxical vocal fold movement. *Am J Speech Lang Pathol.* 2008;17(4):327–334.
28. Giliberto JP, Dibildox D, Merati A. Unilateral laryngoscopic findings associated with response to gabapentin in patients with chronic cough. *JAMA Otolaryngol Head Neck Surg.* 2017;143(11):1081–1085.
29. Hartley NA, Thibeault SL. Systemic hydration: relating science to clinical practice in vocal health. *J Voice.* 2014;28(5):652.e1–652.e20.
30. Sivasankar M, Leydon C. The role of hydration in vocal fold physiology. *Curr Opin Otolaryngol Head Neck Surg.* 2010;18(3):171–175.
31. Blager FB, Gay ML, Wood RP. Voice therapy techniques adapted to treatment of habit cough: a pilot study. *J Commun Disord.* 1988;21(5):393–400.
32. Steinhauer K, McDonald Klimek M, Estill J. *The Estill Voice Model: Theory Translation.* Pittsburgh, PA: Estill Voice International; 2017.
33. Mathers-Schmidt BA. Paradoxical vocal fold motion: a tutorial on a complex disorder and the speech-language pathologist's role. *Am J Speech Lang Pathol.* 2001;10:111–125.
34. Wilson Arboleda BM, Frederick AL. Considerations for maintenance of postural alignment for voice production. *J Voice.* 2008;22(1):90–99.
35. Morrow B, Brink J, Grace S, Pritchard L, Lupton-Smith A. The effect of positioning and diaphragmatic breathing exercises on respiratory muscle activity in people with chronic obstructive pulmonary disease. *South Afr J Physiother.* 2016;72(1):315.
36. Solow B, Sandham A. Cranio-cervical posture: a factor in the development and function of the dentofacial structures. *Eur J Orthod.* 2002;24(5):447–456.

37. Chaitow L, Bradley D, Gilbert C, Bartley J, Peters D. *Recognizing and Treating Breathing Disorders: A Multidisciplinary Approach*. New York, NY: Elsevier; 2014.
38. Courtney R. The importance of correct breathing for raising healthy good looking children. *J Aust Tradit Med Soc.* 2013;19(1):20–27.
39. Han J, Park S, Kim Y, Choi Y, Lyu H. Effects of forward head posture on forced vital capacity and respiratory muscles activity. *J Phys Ther Sci.* 2016;28(1):128–131.
40. Dimitriadis Z, Kapreli E, Strimpakos N, Oldham J. Pulmonary function of patients with chronic neck pain: a spirometry study. *Respir Care.* 2014;59(4): 543–549.
41. Gilman M, Johns MM. The effect of head position and/or stance on the self-perception of phonatory effort. *J Voice.* 2017;31(1):131.e1–131.e4.
42. Cardoso R, Lumini-Oliveira J, Meneses RF. Associations between posture, voice, and dysphonia: a systematic review. *J Voice.* Published online: Oct. 11, 2017.
43. Rees CJ, Henderson AH, Belafsky PC. Postviral vagal neuropathy. *Ann Otol Rhinol Laryngol.* 2009;118(4):247–252.
44. Mathers-Schmidt BA, Brilla LR. Inspiratory muscle training in exercise-induced paradoxical vocal fold motion. *J Voice.* 2005;19(4):635–644.
45. Miller WR, Rollnick S. *Motivational Interviewing: Helping People Change.* New York/London: Guilford; 2012.
46. Behrman A. Facilitating behavioral change in voice therapy: the relevance of motivational interviewing. *Am J Speech Lang Pathol.* 2006;15(3):215–225.
47. Crawley BK, Murry T, Sulica L. Injection augmentation for chronic cough. *J Voice.* 2015;29(6):763–767.
48. Kang CH, Hentz JG, Lott DG. Muscle tension dysphagia: symptomology and theoretical framework. *Otolaryngol Head Neck Surg.* 2016;155(5):837–842.
49. Elkins GR, Barabasz AF, Council JR, Spiegel D. Advancing research and practice: the Revised APA Division 30 definition of hypnosis. *Am J Clin Hypn.* 2015;57(4):378–385.
50. Hammond DC, American Society of Clinical Hypnosis. *Hypnotic Induction Suggestion.* Chicago, IL: American Society of Clinical Hypnosis; 1998.
51. Anbar RD, Hall HR. Childhood habit cough treated with self-hypnosis. *J Pediatr.* 2004;144(2):213–217.
52. Roy N, Bless DM, Heisey D, Ford CN. Manual circumlaryngeal therapy for functional dysphonia: an evaluation of short- and long-term treatment outcomes. *J Voice.* 1997;11(3):321–331.
53. Aronson AE. *The Manual Laryngeal Muscle Tension Reduction Technique*. Rochester, MN: Mentor Seminars; 1997.
54. Roy N, Peterson EA, Pierce JL, Smith ME, Houtz DR. Manual laryngeal reposturing as a primary approach for mutational falsetto. *Laryngoscope.* 2017;127(3): 645–650.
55. Diniz LR, Nesi J Curi AC, Martins W. Qualitative evaluation of osteopathic manipulative therapy in a patient with gastroesophageal reflux disease: a brief report. *J Am Osteopath Assoc.* 2014;114(3):180–188.
56. Walt Fritz, 12/26/2017, personal communication
57. Michele Fava, MC-S. 1/15/2018, personal communication
58. Hagman C, Janson C, Emtner M. A comparison between patients with dysfunctional breathing and patients with asthma. *Clin Respir J.* 2008;2(2):86–91.
59. Boulding R, Stacey R, Niven R, Fowler SJ. Dysfunctional breathing: a review of the literature and proposal for classification. *Eur Respir Rev.* 2016;25(141):287–294.

60. Balkissoon R, Kenn K. Asthma: vocal cord dysfunction (VCD) and other dysfunctional breathing disorders. *Semin Respir Crit Care Med.* 2012;33(6):595–605.
61. Barker N, Everard ML. Getting to grips with "dysfunctional breathing." *Paediatr Respir Rev.* 2015;16(1):53–61.
62. Courtney R, van Dixhoorn J, Greenwood KM, Anthonissen EL. Medically unexplained dyspnea: partly moderated by dysfunctional (thoracic dominant) breathing pattern. *J Asthma.* 2011;48(3):259–265.
63. Mitchell AJ, Bacon CJ, Moran RW. Reliability and determinants of Self-Evaluation of Breathing Questionnaire (SEBQ) score: a symptoms-based measure of dysfunctional breathing. *Appl Psychophysiol Biofeedback.* 2016;41(1):111–120.
64. Courtney R. Breathing training for dysfunctional breathing in asthma: taking a multidimensional approach. *ERJ Open Res.* 2017;3(4).
65. CliftonSmith T, Rowley J. Breathing pattern disorders and physiotherapy: inspiration for our profession. *Physical Therapy Reviews.* 2013;16(1):75–86.
66. Thomas M, McKinley RK, Freeman E, Foy C, Price D. The prevalence of dysfunctional breathing in adults in the community with and without asthma. *Prim Care Respir J.* 2005;14(2):78–82.
67. Thomas M, McKinley RK, Freeman E, Foy C. Prevalence of dysfunctional breathing in patients treated for asthma in primary care: cross-sectional survey. *BMJ.* 2001;322(7294):1098–1100.
68. Cowley DS, Roy-Byrne PP. Hyperventilation and panic disorder. *Am J Med.* 1987;83(5):929–937.
69. Stanton AE, Vaughn P, Carter R, Bucknall CE. An observational investigation of dysfunctional breathing and breathing control therapy in a problem asthma clinic. *J Asthma.* 2008;45(9):758–765.
70. Robson A. Dyspnoea, hyperventilation and functional cough: a guide to which tests help sort them out. *Breathe (Sheff).* 2017;13(1):45–50.
71. Courtney R. A multi-dimensional model of dysfunctional breathing and integrative breathing therapy—commentary on the functions of breathing and its dysfunctions and their relationship to breathing therapy. *J Yoga Phys Ther.* 2016;06(04):257.
72. Courtney R, Cohen M. Investigating the claims of Konstantin Buteyko, M.D, Ph.D.: the relationship of breath holding time to end-tidal CO2 and other proposed measures of dysfunctional breathing. *J Altern Complement Med.* 2008; 14(2):115–123.
73. Jack S, Rossiter HB, Warburton CJ, Whipp BJ. Behavioral influences and physiological indices of ventilatory control in subjects with idiopathic hyperventilation. *Behav Modif.* 2003;27(5):637–652.
74. Courtney R, van Dixhoorn J, Cohen M. Evaluation of breathing pattern: comparison of a Manual Assessment of Respiratory Motion (MARM) and respiratory induction plethysmography. *Appl Psychophysiol Biofeedback.* 2008;33(2):91–100.
75. Hoyte FC. Vocal cord dysfunction. *Immunol Allergy Clin North Am.* 2013;33(1): 1–22.
76. Parker JM, Berg BW. Prevalence of hyperventilation in patients with vocal cord dysfunction. *Chest.* 2002;122(4):185.
77. Thomas M, McKinley RK, Freeman E, Foy C, Prodger P, Price D. Breathing retraining for dysfunctional breathing in asthma: a randomised controlled trial. *Thorax.* 2003;58(2):110–115.

78. West JB. *Respiratory Physiology: The Essentials*. Philadelphia, PA: Wolters Kluwer/ Lippincott Williams Wilkins; 2014.
79. Cowie RL, Conley DP, Underwood MF, Reader PG. A randomised controlled trial of the Buteyko technique as an adjunct to conventional management of asthma. *Respir Med*. 2008;102(5):726–732.
80. Cooper S, Oborne J, Newton S, et al. Effect of two breathing exercises (Buteyko and pranayama) in asthma: a randomised controlled trial. *Thorax*. 2003;58(8): 674–679.
81. McHugh P, Duncan B, Houghton F. Buteyko breathing technique and asthma in children: a case series. *N Z Med J*. 2006;119(1234):U1988.
82. Jenkins D. The oxygen advantage: the simple, scientifically proven breathing techniques for a healthier, slimmer, faster, and fitter you. *Cranio*. 2016;34(2): 139–140
83. Lumb AB, Nunn JF. *Nunn's Applied Respiratory Physiology*. Oxford, UK: Elsevier Butterworth-Heinemann; 2005.
84. Vertigan AE, Theodoros DG, Gibson PG, Winkworth AL. Voice and upper airway symptoms in people with chronic cough and paradoxical vocal fold movement. *J Voice*. 2007;21(3):361–383.
85. Hallani M, Wheatley JR, Amis TC. Enforced mouth breathing decreases lung function in mild asthmatics. *Respirology*. 2008;13(4):553–558.
86. Shturman-Ellstein R, Zeballos RJ, Buckley JM, Souhrada JF. The beneficial effect of nasal breathing on exercise-induced bronchoconstriction. *Am Rev Respir Dis*. 1978;118(1):65–73.
87. Kim EJ, Choi JH, Kim KW, et al. The impacts of open-mouth breathing on upper airway space in obstructive sleep apnea: 3-D MDCT analysis. *Eur Arch Otorhinolaryngol*. 2011;268(4):533–539.
88. Brown RP, Gerbarg PL. Sudarshan Kriya yogic breathing in the treatment of stress, anxiety, and depression: part I-neurophysiologic model. *J Altern Complement Med*. 2005;11(1):189–201.
89. Courtney R. (2011). *Dysfunctional breathing: its parameters, measurement and relevance* [PhD thesis].
90. Han J, Zhu Y, Li S, et al. The language of medically unexplained dyspnea. *Chest*. 2008;133(4):961–968.

9

A TREATMENT PARADIGM FOR REFRACTORY CHRONIC COUGH

Putting It All Together in a Quaternary Cough Referral Practice

Thomas L. Carroll

INTRODUCTION

The chapters of this book were chosen to clearly establish the multidisciplinary nature of the treatment for chronic cough. It would be ideal for every chronic cough patient to see a seasoned chronic cough clinical team on first presentation, but this is not realistic due to reasons of geography, cost, and patient convenience. As discussed in Chapter 1, most cases are managed by the first physician the patient approaches. The etiology of the cough is usually conquered by the initial physician if it is one of the three common causes of cough: asthma, reflux, or upper airway cough syndrome (allergy and sinus). The minority of cases will require specialty visits to rule in and/or rule out etiologies for chronic cough. An ever-smaller portion of cases will eventually end up in a subspecialty center that has an expert team to evaluate and treat the most refractory cases of chronic cough. Subspecialty voice, airway, and swallowing centers ("voice centers") composed of fellowship-trained laryngologists and cough- and voice-specialized speech-language pathologists often represent this "bottom of the funnel" subspecialty practice, with the treating physician leading the data collection, interpreting prior medical testing results, and directing further workup and treatment.

Any specialist can serve as the knowledgeable point person in a health system or community to direct further workup and care for chronic cough patients. However, most patients who present to voice centers with intractable chronic cough have previously been evaluated and treated unsuccessfully, or at a minimum incompletely, medically and surgically by various pulmonologists, allergists and immunologists, gastroenterologists, primary care providers, and other general or subspecialty-trained otolaryngologists for months, if not years. The reader should understand that the term "voice center" will be used for convenience to define the teritary or quaternary clinician and their team of chronic cough treatment providers, but the reader should also understand that this clinician may not always be a laryngologist or otolaryngologist. This chapter will focus on the final pathway for evaluating and treating chronic cough patients who may have already been seen by multiple providers.

A FLEXIBLE INITIAL APPROACH TO A NEW PATIENT

Chronic cough is a symptom, not a diagnosis. There is almost universally a discoverable etiology for chronic cough, potentially multifactorial, and when all tests and treatments are completed by a willing patient, an idiopathic or unknown cause for the chronic cough will rarely be the diagnosis. It would be ideal to have an algorithm to follow for refractory chronic cough patients. However, patients do not always easily fit into the algorithm, nor do they have only one etiology contributing to their cough. Patients have often tried and failed multiple medications prescribed one or more times by multiple providers at various doses without a clear pattern of escalation or substitution. Similarly, reasons for initiating or terminating the treatments are often vague or fall into the category of "it just didn't help." Most patients have been seen by several physicians along the road to the voice center team and have often had many empiric trials of medications for chronic cough and repeated testing, including tests for pulmonary, gastroenterological, and sinonasal etiologies for the cough. Patients express feelings of hopelessness when they are referred to their ultimate chronic cough care team based on the lack of success leading up to the visit. It is often paramount to give them hope at the first visit or at least reveal what can be further evaluated and tried that has not already been done (if anything).

It is not unusual to meet a patient who has been on multiple steroid inhalers for years despite having normal pulmonary function testing (PFT), has never had bronchodilator improvement on PFTs, and has never been offered bronchoprovocation testing such as methacholine challenge testing to rule out asthma (see Chapter 2). It is also not unusual to meet refractory chronic cough patients who have already undergone sinonasal surgery without improvement in their postnasal drip symptoms, despite never having had chronic sinusitis documented. These patients may have met criteria for septoplasty (straightening of the nasal septum to improve breathing), but due to the lack of complete workup for other etiologies of chronic cough, the patients received surgery that did not fix the chronic cough complaint for which they presented. It is not uncommon for chronic cough patients to report partial or temporary relief with topical and systemic steroid treatments. Steroids are nondiscriminatory in treating inflammation and can work on inflamed tissues of the oropharynx, nasopharynx, larynx, and airways regardless of the underlying etiology of the inflammation.

A definitive reflux workup is also often incomplete when chronic cough patients present to a voice center. Patients are often told they do not have reflux or, more commonly, that reflux is not causing the chronic cough because their reflux medication and normal upper gastroesophageal endoscopy (EGD) are sufficient to rule out reflux as a cause of their chronic cough. However, acid suppression has been shown to not control physiologic reflux (see Chapter 4).[1] Our understanding of how the digestive enzyme pepsin is the probable culprit in causing laryngopharyngeal reflux (LPR) symptoms is maturing, as is our understanding of what happens when we eliminate reflux and not just acid from the laryngopharynx. Chronic cough often improves after antireflux surgery in patients with chronic cough and positive pharyngeal reflux events demonstrated on impedance probes that cover the entire esophagus and span the upper esophageal sphincter (UES) to the oropharynx (hypopharyngeal-esophageal multichannel intraluminal impedance with dual pH, "HEMII-pH").[2] We can now better understand the pathophysiology of LPR, its role in chronic cough and thus more clearly explain to our patients how traditional modalities (prior gold standards such as dual pH probes) for diagnosing gastroesophageal reflux disease (GERD) are inadequate to rule out reflux as the cause of chronic cough.[3] Patients routinely present with normal 24-hour dual probe pH tests and, more recently, normal pharyngeal ph-metry testing results (Restech® Dx-pH probe, Respiratory Technology Corp, San Diego, CA) and dual pH with impedance that only detects liquid events up to 17 cm above the LES and not above the UES as is the case with HEMII-pH.

As discussed in Chapter 4, GERD and LPR are different presentations of a common underlying phenomenon: the physiologic retrograde movement of gastric contents superiorly. Reflux testing with HEMII-pH has the ability to rule in LPR as an etiology for refractory chronic cough and characterize the acidity or lack thereof in the refluxate.[2,4] High-resolution esophageal manometry (HRM) is also a missing component in the workup of the chronic cough patient. Many patients do not have true reflux from the stomach; rather, they present with chronic cough or other LPR symptoms due to comorbid issues from esophageal dysmotility that lead to direct LPR changes in the laryngopharynx or generate cough through vagally mediated mechanisms form within the esophagus (see Chapter 7).

Due to the breadth of knowledge that must be mastered by most primary care clinicians, general pulmonologists, gastroenterologists, and otolaryngologists, simple algorithms to work through a new chronic cough patient are of value. Figure 9–1 is an algorithm that should aid the front line of treating clinicians.[5]

This algorithm is not realistic and is often impossible to work through in the quaternary referral voice center. Adhering to this and "reinventing the wheel" with every patient leads to time and money wasted, both personal and in health care dollars, for patients who have already been on a long road with a difficult symptom. Collecting previous records, synthesizing the data, and deciding on what options remain for the refractory chronic cough patient is often performed and then options for next steps are determined. If work with a SLP who specializes in cough suppression strategies has never been pursued, this is often prescribed at the first visit to the voice center (see Chapter 8). In addition to the lack of SLP involvement in the management of a patient with refractory chronic cough, the most common omissions from the workup for underlying causes of chronic cough in the author's experience include: bronchoprovocation challenge testing (eg, methacholine challenge testing), HEMII-pH testing, and, in patients with meal-associated coughing, videofluoroscopic swallow studies (VFSS) or flexible endoscopic evaluation of swallowing (FEES) testing.

A few recent papers have addressed the costs associated with the inappropriate, unnecessary, and/or unrelenting treatments and workup for LPR. It appears the health care system could save billions of dollars annually if PPIs were not empirically prescribed for all patients with LPR symptoms, including chronic cough. When considering patients who have been worked up for extraesophageal symptoms of reflux, a study by Francis et al looked at 281 patients, half of whom had cough as their complaint.[6] They found the overall cost per patient improvement (including Medicare costs for diagnosis, treatment, and unnecessary medications, etc) to be $13,700 per patient, most of which came from the prescription of proton-pump inhibitor (PPI) medications. Their initial annual direct cost was $5,154 for the workup of these patients, 5.6 times higher than patients with classic GERD. These data reinforce the trial and error method occurring in the workup and treatment (often empiric trials of PPIs) of chronic cough patients. The overall estimated annual cost in the United States of treating LPR is above $50 billion.[6]

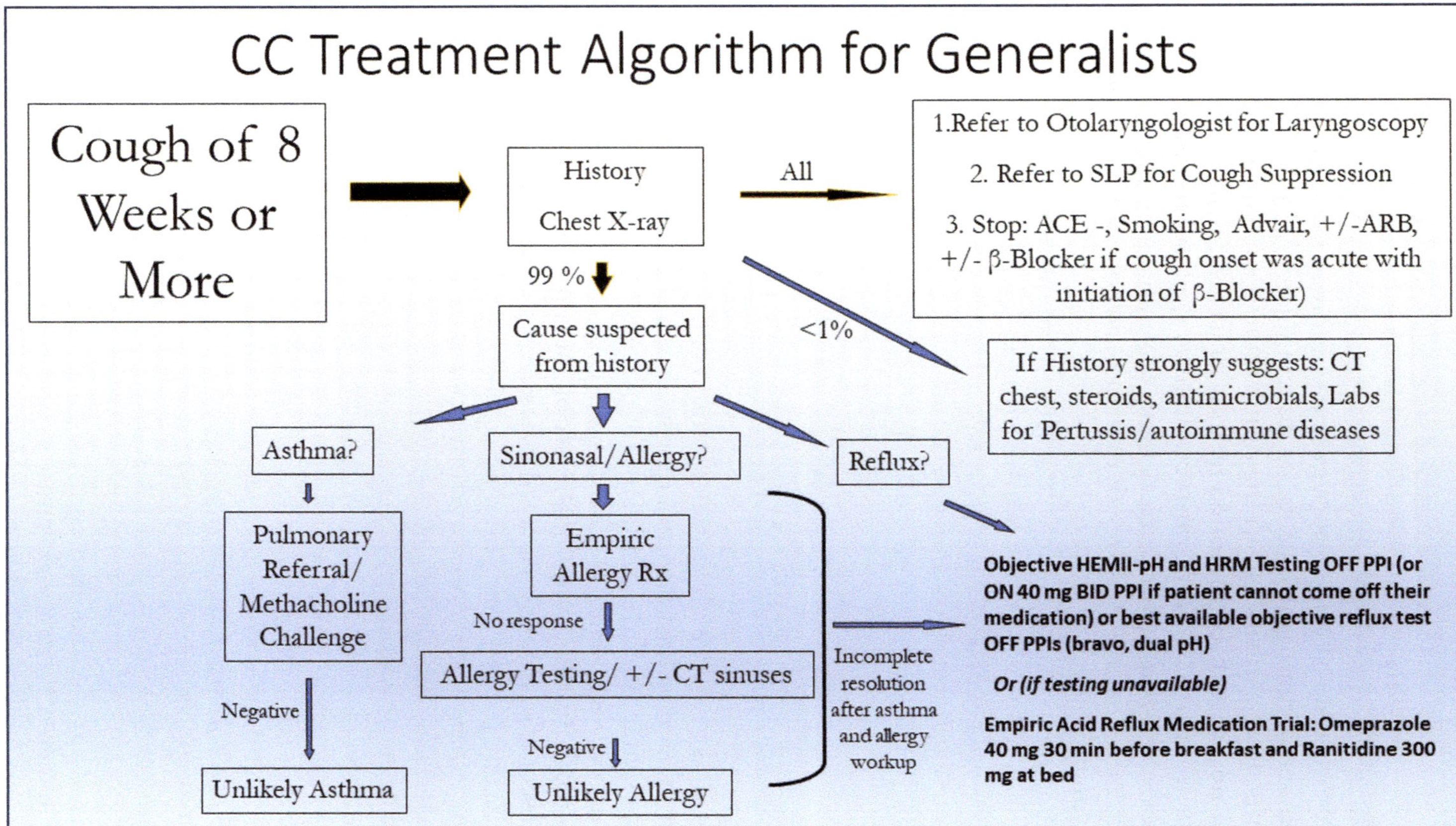

Figure 9–1. The basic chronic cough treatment algorithm (inspired by Pratter et al.[5]). An initial treatment algorithm for treating clinicians on the front lines of chronic cough. This is not ideal for the refractory chronic cough patient who has seen multiple providers and has already had multiple tests and treatments. It is not efficient in these cases because a quaternary chronic cough referral center clinician will have more clinical acumen and can often work in a more efficient and cost-saving manner outside this fixed pathway.

More recently, a study by Carroll et al used the Francis et al study's cost estimates to determine if up-front impedance with dual-pH testing could decrease the cost burden in the reflux workup of patients with LPR.[7] The Carroll study reported an estimated 40% average cost savings over empiric high-dose PPI medication trials. With PPIs being the primary driver of cost to the healthcare system and with more data suggesting potential deleterious side effects of PPI use, up-front reflux testing makes sense.[8] Many centers (and thus patients) do not have access to HEMII-pH testing, thus the ability to perform a 24-hour reflux test that evaluates acid and nonacid refluxed stomach contents to and above the UES. Using clinical acumen and positive predictive value in the face of patient-reported symptoms beyond chronic cough, more traditional tests for reflux such as capsule pH-metry (BRAVO™ Reflux Testing System, Medtronic Inc, Minneapolis, MN) or dual pH probes may be worth exploring first before prescribing PPIs. If up-front, acid-only reflux testing is unrevealing, it may at least prevent unnecessary PPI prescriptions and lead to further referral to a center where HEMII-pH testing is available for some chronic cough patients.

ASKING FOR THE RIGHT HELP AT THE RIGHT TIME

Instead of an algorithm, the diagrammatic approach to the refractory chronic cough patient who has already had a thorough workup by numerous other providers and who has tried prior medical or surgical therapies is more akin to a treatment "wheel" (Figure 9–2). The quaternary chronic cough clinician sits with the patient at the center of the wheel, and all available unexplored options reside at the end of the spokes leading to and from the center. The treating clinician can pull any and all diagnostic and therapeutic options back from the rim individually or in tandem. Depending on the quaternary clinician's specialty, the spokes of the wheel will vary. For example, if a pulmonologist is the lead, a laryngologist would be at the end of one of the spokes and vice versa. For many patients, the number of spokes will be few due to their prior workup, and thus the potential for improvement is closer at hand. Some patients have had a partial or incomplete workup in numerous areas, and more spokes of the wheel will potentially need to be explored. Any missing pieces, especially of the prior pulmonary and sinonasal workup, are identified, as are treatments that can be offered for chronic cough beyond the big three etiologies. It is important to know what options remain for the patient (ie, they have already had a good neuromodulator medication trial, or they underwent vocal fold augmentation for a known paresis).

Clinical experience and positive predictive value of which etiology is causing the chronic cough will typically direct the order in which patients explore different spokes on the wheel. Etiologies with malignant potential

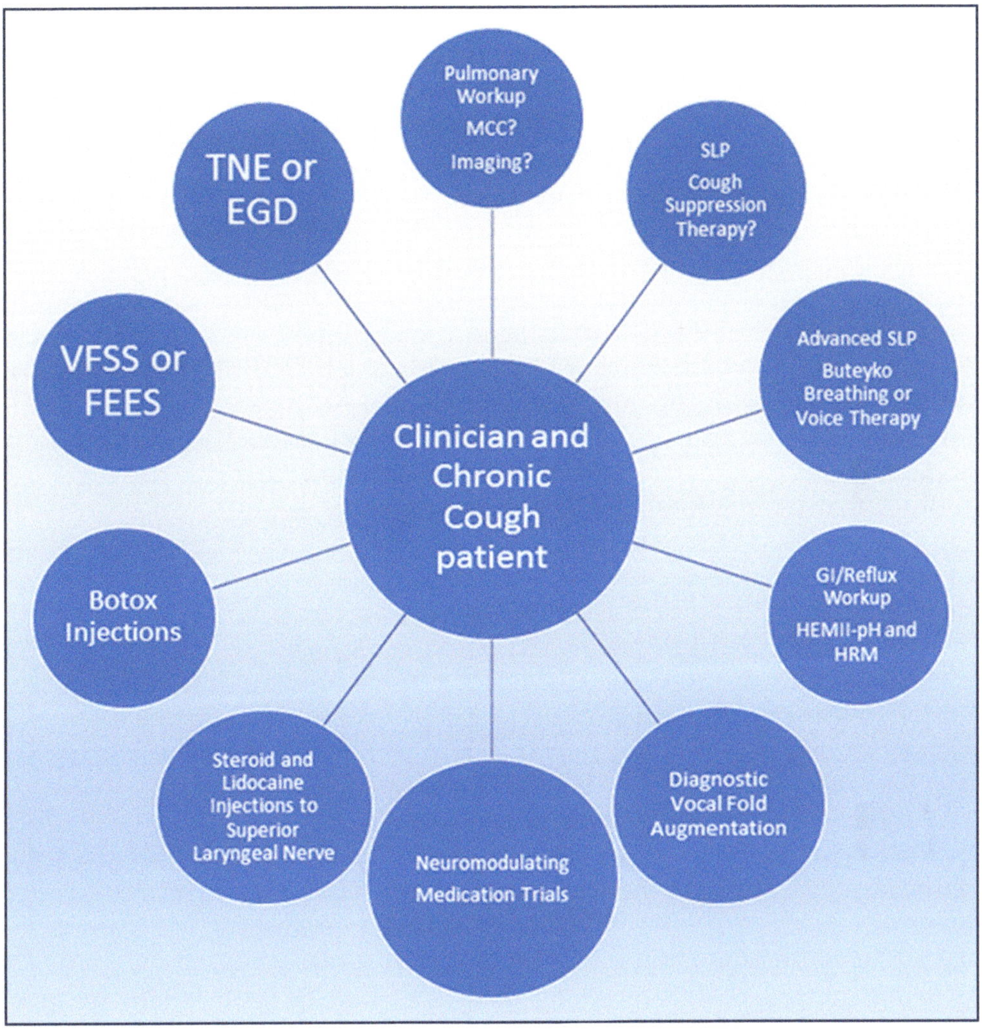

Figure 9–2. The refractory chronic cough wheel. With the patient and quaternary clinician at the center, clinical judgment and patient history guide which spokes of the wheel deserve exploration. The patient is sent "out" the spokes to another specialist, diagnostic, or treatment option then returns "in" for reassessment and further consideration if necessary.

are always explored first, or at least in tandem with the highest nonmalignant potential etiology, especially in smokers. Cancers of the esophagus, airway, lung, and head and neck are always on the radar of the quaternary chronic cough clinician. These concerns seem obvious, but they can easily be overlooked—for example, if the chronic cough patient is a smoker and has yet to see a pulmonologist, or if the patient has solid food dysphagia and a barium swallow, or better yet an EGD, has not been performed in a prior heavy smoker. Chronic cough in the face of persistent hoarseness is often accompanied by benign vocal fold changes, but laryngoscopy is required in patients with persistent hoarseness of 4 weeks or more to rule out laryngeal or other mucosal malignancies of the head and neck. In smokers the 4-week waiting period is ignored when there is no other reason for the voice change (concurrent upper respiratory infection, etc).[9] Chronic cough in the face of unilateral middle ear effusion, unremitting nasal obstruction and recurrent epistaxis requires nasopharyngoscopy and nasal endoscopy before treating empirically to rule out sinonasal tumors.

Despite voice centers seeing patients who have typically experienced multiple tests and treatments, the big three causes of chronic cough cannot be forgotten, as they have often been incompletely explored. The most common incomplete workup is in the reflux category, but confirmation of normal chest imaging, no angiotensin-converter enzyme inhibitor use (ACE inhibitors such as lisinopril), allergy testing and medication trial results, and sinonasal imaging are nearly universally required. It can't be repeated enough that the etiology of a chronic cough can be multifactorial, and it can't be said enough times that a treatment failure may be a partial success. The voice center should work to evaluate all previous partial successes as they relate to the time course in the patient's chronic cough history. Trying to determine if multiple prior diagnoses can be tied to one underlying pathology is always the goal, but is not always proven. The two common underlying themes that can affect the lungs, larynx, and sinonasal mucosa are the unified airway (see Chapter 3) and pepsin-mediated reflux disease (see Chapter 5).

Again, most patients who present to a voice center have typically had the unified airway thoroughly evaluated and treated; this leaves the nonacid reflux etiology with the most room for impact and discovery. For patients who have been appropriately worked up and treated for pulmonary and sinonasal etiologies, the initial recommendation for patients in whom reflux is suspected is HEMII-pH testing with HRM. Because dysmotility, nonacidic high esophageal (just below the UES), or pharyngeal reflux events are often missed without HEMII-pH and HRM testing, these tests can and, because of cost savings, should be performed before trying further acid suppression or centrally acting neuromodulating medications for presumed postviral vagal neuropathy (PVVN) (see Chapter 6). If HEMII-pH and HRM testing is not readily available (eg, months' wait before testing date, as can be the case) or the patient is truly miserable from their cough, it is reasonable to offer high-dose acid suppression trials or neuromodulator medication trials based on the patient history if these have not previously been offered.

It cannot be stressed enough to universally recommend a chronic cough–knowledgeable treating SLP in your practice or community who can work with a patient on cough suppression techniques as discussed in Chapter 8. In the voice center, not only are basic cough suppression techniques taught to patients but, for the patient who has talking as a trigger or other vocal fold pathology that may be affected by ongoing cough, voice therapy is also prescribed. The voice therapist is invaluable in the treatment of chronic cough patients. Education on laryngeal hygiene alone is something most physicians cannot offer. More advanced techniques such as Buteyko breathing are placed on an individual spoke of the wheel because not all patients require this level and intensity of training.[10–11] However, Buteyko breathing should be considered as an adjunct treatment that can significantly decrease chronic cough and improve concomitant breathing complaints such as paradoxical vocal fold motion disorder (see Chapters 8 and 10).

FINE TUNING THE DIAGNOSIS AND TREATMENT

As mentioned above, bronchoprovocation challenge, HEMII-pH, and VFSS testing are anecdotally the most commonly overlooked tests in patients with excellent prior chronic cough workups, in the author's experience. Bronchoprovocation testing is not commonly performed in the community and can aid in ruling out asthma as a cause of cough in patients who do not respond to bronchodilators (see Chapter 2). HEMII-pH testing may require a tertiary referral, and has often been supplanted due to convenience by a test that cannot evaluate nonacid reflux throughout the esophagus and up at and above the UES. Patients are never excited about repeating a test that involves a wire in their nose for 24 hours, but a frank conversation about why this test may be revealing is always worthwhile. In a patient with few to no other options and who refuses a repeat 24-hour HEMII-pH probe, an empiric trial of alginate therapy (ie, Gaviscon Advance liquid, Reckitt Benckiser, United Kingdom) is offered.[12] Alginate therapy is also offered before referral for antireflux surgery in patients with positive nonacid reflux on HEMII-pH testing (see Chapter 4). VFSS or FEES testing is always worthwhile in patients with meal-associated chronic cough (see Chapter 7) and otherwise normal neurolaryngeal function on flexible laryngoscopy.

It is important to emphasize that demonstrating an undiscovered etiology for chronic cough to a patient with years, if not decades, of symptoms is half the battle. The most common example of this is in reflux patients who have been told they do not have reflux. Demonstrating nonacid reflux that the patient cannot feel/detect on their own is the impetus for many to finally follow through with diet and lifestyle changes as well as treatment compliance in an effort to improve their symptoms. At a minimum, patients stop their endless search for why they cough and focus on any and all options to treat it. Alginate therapy often improves chronic cough in the right (albeit compliant) patient, but due to the regimen of needing to take this medicine four to five times daily, many will try other chronic cough treatments in addition to diet and lifestyle modification. Neuromodulator trials can and do work in the face of known reflux.

This is likely because the insult to the vagus nerve that caused sphincter dysfunction, dysmotility, and decreased gastric emptying (thus real reflux) also caused the patient's vocal fold paresis and sensory issues. If a patient has a normal esophagus on endoscopy and does not respond to or cannot tolerate alginates, neuromodulator medications are a good step before recommending surgery for reflux (see the following).

Final options for patients who have explored the majority of the spokes of the wheel involve less scientifically studied interventions or invasive surgical procedures that are both diagnostic and therapeutic. Injection augmentation for glottic insufficiency to improve vocal fold closure in the face of subtle air loss from the vocal folds during phonation (typically from vocal fold paresis, thinning/atrophy, or scarring) has shown potential to improve chronic cough in the right patient (see Chapter 10). Steroid and lidocaine injections to the area of the superior laryngeal nerve as it enters the thyrohyoid space above the larynx, as well as botulinum toxin injections to the vocal fold adductor muscles, are final treatment options in patients who have tried and failed other treatments, even in the setting of proven reflux or allergies (see Chapter 10).

Antireflux surgery, most often Nissen fundoplication (Nissen), is indicated for the right chronic cough patient, but what defines the right chronic cough patient is often the patient themselves. Anecdotally, 1 in 100 patients seen in the author's practice will pursue and complete antireflux surgery. Having known pharyngeal events or an elevated number of events at the UES does not mean the patient will or should be referred for Nissen. On the contrary, some patients present to a voice center after years under the care of a gastroenterologist who will not recommend Nissen despite persistent regurgitation. This is often because the patient's EGD is normal and PPIs are controlling the acid component of the reflux. These chronic cough patients are often good candidates to refer for Nissen because they desperately want relief and are willing to take the associated risks. Most chronic cough patients must try everything possible before considering Nissen. If quality of life remains affected by the cough despite exhausting all other treatments in the face of known hypopharyngeal reflux events, a patient may choose to consult with a general or thoracic surgeon. Other forms of antireflux surgery exist but are not as well reported for outcomes in cases of refractory chronic cough.[13–15] Nissen involves reducing a hiatal hernia if present and wrapping the top of the stomach around the bottom of the esophagus, thus tightening the area of the lower esophageal sphincter and turning it into a one-way valve.

Nissen is life changing for most chronic cough patients in both good and bad ways. For those chronic cough patients diagnosed with LPR through HEMII-pH testing and HRM, the success rate of Nissen to relieve cough appears excellent, even when the reflux events did not correlate specifically with cough events during testing.[16–18] The downside to Nissen is typically transient dysphagia and the inability to burp or vomit. Bronchial thermoplasty is an option for patients with refractory chronic cough in the face of asthma (see Chapter 2).[19] Both antireflux surgery and bronchial thermoplasty may make the patient worse before they get better; patients must be counseled appropriately by the treating surgeon or interventional pulmonologist.

In conclusion, the refractory chronic cough patient who eventually finds a voice center should expect all prior treatment and diagnostic information to be synthesized, a cough- and dyspnea-knowledgeable SLP to become involved in their care, and all additional spokes on the wheel to be explored as deemed necessary and in the order determined most likely to succeed by the lead clinician. This role does not require a physician, but often involves one. This team leader is often a laryngologist or other otolaryngologist who has an interest in chronic cough and who can easily visualize and evaluate the functions of the larynx with and without stroboscopy.

THINKING OUTSIDE OF THE BOX

Nonacid LPR is the most common cause of chronic cough in the experience of the author in patients presenting to a quaternary voice center. It is not uncommon for patients to present having had other reflux testing but not HEMII-pH with HRM. While it seems like such a small piece of additional information to get impedance information at and above the UES, the results do make a difference. Dysmotility can be a contributor to the patient's chronic cough picture, and HRM reveals this routinely as a potential contributing etiology (especially in cases of achalasia with no meaningful peristalsis). It is amazing to see the transformation from hopelessness to hope and the increased success rates in patients who have been told there was no known etiology for their chronic cough; they are now motivated by potentially treatable etiologies of chronic cough. Alginate therapy has become a mainstay in the initial treatment of nonacid reflux in patients proven to have nonacid reflux on HEMII-pH testing.

When presented with a new chronic cough patient in any setting —primary, tertiary, or quaternary—data synthesis cannot be emphasized enough. One should take a step back and the spokes of the wheel need to be evaluated. When to ask for help depends on the individual clinician's skill set and comfort level, but it is shocking to see how many patients go through trial and error as well as presumed diagnoses, such as asthma from their primary care provider, or LPR from their otolaryngologist, without any objective testing. LPR does not cause all symptoms in the larynx, including chronic cough, and it is right to question a long-standing LPR diagnosis. This is especially true in a patient diagnosed by an otolaryngologist who did not use stroboscopy to look for other vocal fold pathologies or who has been treated with PPIs, without success, for years. A presumed asthma diagnosis is also a common stumbling block for patients and clinicians. After decades on inhalers the diagnosis is often hard to consider as wrong or incomplete. Children reflux, and patients diagnosed with asthma as children who have not had objective testing in adulthood, deserve this. It may have been reflux injury to the larynx or lungs and may never have been true asthma to start with. Along the same vein, idiopathic pulmonary fibrosis triggers alarms for the senior author, especially in patients with concomitant, uncontrolled GERD symptoms such as acid brash or regurgitation.

Although this chapter promotes undiagnosed LPR as a common etiology for persistent and refractory chronic cough, it cannot be emphasized enough that a team approach is needed. Not all patients have a thorough workup as they present to a voice center. The ability for the voice center lead clinician to refer to SLP, pulmonary, allergy, sinonasal, and gastroenterology colleagues when pieces of the story are missing or incomplete is paramount. No one clinician can treat chronic cough in a silo, nor should they.

TAKE-HOME POINTS

- Subspecialty voice centers, composed of fellowship-trained laryngologists and cough- and voice-specialized speech-language pathologists, often represent this bottom of the funnel subspecialty practice in the treatment of chronic cough; however, this is not always the case in all health systems and hospitals, and other clinical subspecialists commonly lead chronic cough care teams with similar success.
- Flexibility by the clinician lead in a voice center will allow a more efficient treatment plan than sticking to a fixed algorithm. The cough wheel should be considered when evaluating what has been done for a patient leading up to the initial visit and what remains possible to help diagnose or treat their chronic cough.
- Bronchoprovocation challenge testing, objective swallow testing (VFSS and FEES), and reflux testing that incorporates dual pH and impedance from the lower sphincter to above the upper sphincter (HEMII-pH) with high-resolution manometry are the author's most commonly missed elements to the workup of a refractory chronic cough patient. They may not all be needed, but the

patient history should direct if any or all are needed to aid in the diagnosis.

- Nonacid reflux is the most common cause of chronic cough in the author's quaternary referral center.

REFERENCES

1. Blonski W, Vela MF, Castell DO. Comparison of reflux frequency during prolonged multichannel intraluminal impedance and pH monitoring on and off acid suppression therapy. *J Clin Gastroenterol.* 2009;43(9):816.
2. Hoppo T, Sanz AF, Nason KS, et al. How much pharyngeal exposure is "normal"? Normative data for laryngopharyngeal reflux events using hypopharyngeal multichannel intraluminal impedance (HMII). *J Gastrointest Surg.* 2012;16(1):16–25.
3. Samuels TL, Johnston N. Pepsin as a marker of extraesophageal reflux. *Ann Otol Rhinol Laryngol.* 2010;119(3):203.
4. Ummarino D, Vandermeulen L, Roosens B, Urbain D, Hauser B, Vandenplas Y. Gastroesophageal reflux evaluation in patients affected by chronic cough: restech versus multichannel intraluminal impedance/pH metry. *Laryngoscope.* 2013;123(4):980–984.
5. Pratter MR, Brightling CE, Boulet LP, Irwin RS. An empiric integrative approach to the management of cough. *Chest.* 2006;129(1):222S–231S.
6. Francis DO, Rymer JA, Slaughter JC, et al. High economic burden of caring for patients with suspected extraesophageal reflux. *Am J Gastroenterol.* 2013;108(6): 905–911.
7. Carroll TL, Werner A, Nahikian K, Dezube A, Roth DF. Rethinking the laryngopharyngeal reflux treatment algorithm: Evaluating an alternate empiric dosing regimen and considering up-front, pH-impedance, and manometry testing to minimize cost in treating suspect laryngopharyngeal reflux disease. *Laryngoscope.* 2017;127:S1–S13.
8. Reimer C. Safety of long-term PPI therapy. *Best Pract Res Clin Gastroenterol.* 2013;27(3):443–454.
9. Stachler RJ, Francis DO, Schwartz SR, et al. Clinical practice guideline: hoarseness (dysphonia)(update). *Otolaryngol Head Neck Surg.* 2018;158(suppl 1): S1–S42.
10. West JB. *Respiratory Physiology: The Essentials.* Philadelphia, PA: Wolters Kluwer/ Lippincott Williams Wilkins; 2014.
11. Cowie RL, Conley DP, Underwood MF, Reader PG. A randomised controlled trial of the Buteyko technique as an adjunct to conventional management of asthma. *Respir Med.* 2008;102(5):726–732.
12. McGlashan JA, Johnstone LM, Sykes J, Strugala V, Dettmar PW. The value of a liquid alginate suspension (Gaviscon Advance) in the management of laryngopharyngeal reflux. *Eur Arch Otorhinolaryngol.* 2009;266(2):243–251.
13. Bell R, Lipham J, Louie B, et al. Laparoscopic magnetic sphincter augmentation versus double-dose proton pump inhibitors for management of moderate-to-

severe regurgitation in GERD: a randomized controlled trial [published online ahead of print July 18, 2018]. *Gastrointest Endosc.* http://www.sciencedirect.com/science/article/pii/S0016510718328487.

14. Rebecchi F, Allaix ME, Cinti L, Nestorović, M, Morino, M. (2018). Comparison of the outcome of laparoscopic procedures for GERD. *Updates Surg*, 1–7.
15. McCarty TR, Itidiare M, Njei B, Rustagi T. Efficacy of transoral incisionless fundoplication for refractory gastroesophageal reflux disease: a systematic review and meta-analysis. *Endoscopy.* 2018;50(07):708–725.
16. Hoppo T, Komatsu Y, Jobe BA. Antireflux surgery in patients with chronic cough and abnormal proximal exposure as measured by hypopharyngeal multichannel intraluminal impedance. *JAMA Surg.* 2013;148(7):608–605.
17. Carroll TL, Nahikian K, Asban A, Wiener D. Nissen fundoplication for laryngopharyngeal reflux after patient selection using dual pH, full column impedance testing: a pilot study. *Ann Otol Rhinol Laryngol.* 2016;125(9):722–728.
18. Komatsu Y, Hoppo T, Jobe BA. Proximal reflux as a cause of adult-onset asthma: the case for hypopharyngeal impedance testing to improve the sensitivity of diagnosis. *JAMA Surg.* 2013;148(1):50–58.
19. Torrego A, Sola I, Munoz AM, et al. Bronchial thermoplasty for moderate or severe persistent asthma in adults. *Cochrane Database Syst Rev.* 2014;(3):CD009910.

10

CHRONIC COUGH: FUTURE DIRECTIONS

Adrianna C. Shembel, Paul E. Kwak, and Milan R. Amin

INTRODUCTION

Coughing is a normal physiological reflex, initiated by receptors within the larynx, to protect the airways below the vocal folds from foreign particulates. The reflex can be activated with any number of exogenous or endogenous stimuli, including, but not limited to, upper respiratory infections, smoking, lung pathology, reflux disorders, postnasal drip, and use of ACE inhibitors.[1–9] When coughing becomes nonproductive, refractory, and persists for more than 3 weeks without known underlying cause (eg, upper respiratory infection), it is referred to as chronic cough.[10,11] Although there may be no known physiological reason or benefit for the cough, chronic cough may be precipitated by a known event such as an upper respiratory infection (URI), or may be present in individuals with asthma or chronic irritant exposure. Episodic symptoms of chronic cough usually start with a tickle or sensation in the larynx or pharynx, which quickly turns into coughing fits that can result in incontinence, lightheadedness, or a syncopic event; these presentations can severely affect quality of life to the point of social isolation and agoraphobia.[12–14] Symptoms may worsen with external (eg, noxious fumes, temperature/weather change, exercise), internal (eg, postnasal drip, GERD/LPR), or psychological (eg, stress, anxiety) triggers. The gold standard for the management of chronic cough is a combination of pharmacological intervention (eg, reflux medication) and behavioral management (ie, cough suppression therapy).

Chronic cough remains a complex clinical entity, in that its symptomatology can vary widely and its underlying mechanisms are not well understood. As such, chronic cough presents special challenges for investigators who seek to understand the multifaceted mechanisms that underlie its clinical presentation, and to find treatments that accordingly address these mechanisms. So far, in this book, the authors have focused on the pathophysiology of cough and the common causes of chronic cough, and have discussed the most relevant treatments as well as the quaternary approach to the complex cough patient. This chapter will focus more on the current translational and clinical research on chronic cough, and novel treatments that are emerging. Some of the concepts are controversial and have not yet been fully developed. However, they form a basis on which current cutting-edge therapies are based.

POTENTIAL UNDERLYING MECHANISMS INVOLVED IN COUGH AND IMPLICATIONS FOR TREATMENT

Potential Mechanisms Underlying Abnormal Glottal Reflexive Responses

Abnormal glottal reflex responses caused by inflammation, viral, mechanical, or chemical factors have long been speculated to underlie mechanisms in chronic cough. Specifically, chronic stimulation of sensory fibers within the larynx are thought to alter laryngeal sensory–motor processes (ie, neuroplasticity) and cause atypical responses for subsequent exposure to typical sensory stimuli.[15] However, this hypothesis has largely remained theoretical, with little in the way of empirical studies on this topic. Fortunately, literature from other medical domains could support this mechanistic theory.

One mechanism underlying chronic cough could be the result of local epithelial inflammation. For example, Taramarcaz and colleagues showed epithelial inflammatory damage suggestive of neural changes with picornavirus, a variant of the common cold, in patients with vocal cord dysfunction, which may predispose these patients to a hypersensitive reflexive response in the larynx.[16] Studies have also shown increases in subepithelial antigens in laryngeal tissue of infants with hyperreactive supraglottic responses.[17,18]

Neuroplastic changes resulting in vagally mediated laryngospasms and apneas secondary to overstimulation of chemoreceptors in the airways have been demonstrated in canine models and infants with exposure to gastric secretions of pH levels less than 2.5.[19,20] Afferent nerves in the respiratory system have been shown to not only stimulate an efferent response to chronic irritation, but to also stimulate a local immune response by recruiting local proinflammatory factors (eg, cytokines). This immune response—known as neurogenic inflammation—causes inflammation and can result in airway remodeling at the peripheral level over time.[21,22]

TRPV1 are receptors that cause inflammatory reactions to the airways when exposed to noxious stimuli. Studies by Couto et al and Chandra et al. demonstrated increased activity of TRPV1 in airway tissue with exposure to capsaicin (the active ingredient in hot peppers). TRPV1 have also been shown to increase vascular permeability for calcium and sodium ions responsible for neural conduction, which may explain the increased vagal motor laryngeal reflex response to irritants (eg, capsaicin) in the airways.[15,18,23,24] Efferent vagal motor response has been associated with increased muscle contraction, increased breathing rate, and decreased breathing depth,[5,16,25–27] which may explain why individuals with chronic cough can be triggered with even mild laryngeal irritation and why patients with this condition typically report trouble "catching their breath."

Cortical Influences in Reflexive Cough Pathways

Van den Bergh and colleagues proposed that chronic cough may have more to do with a Pavlovian-like conditioned response or affective-motivational influences than with direct neuroplastic reflexive changes in the central or peripheral nervous system.[28] Put differently, neural connections do much more than sense foreign particulate or irritation at the epithelial or laryngeal level. Behavioral control and information processing mechanisms (eg, associative experiences, perception, attention, emotional processing, and social context) are integrated with these peripheral sensations. The authors suggest the threshold of laryngeal responsiveness may not be to blame, but rather the interaction of sensations and brain behavior mechanisms that result in hyperreactive laryngeal response in patients with chronic cough.[28] Additionally, laryngeal nerve stimulation studies indicate that hyperactive motor responses result from central processing of afferent stimuli, rather than from changes in sensitivity or altered receptor distribution within the larynx.[20]

A possible clinical correlate of this concept may be habitual cough. Often referred to as "psychogenic cough" or "tic cough," this entity has been described by numerous authors.[16–19] While most of the literature focuses on children, adults commonly demonstrate the clinical features as well. Typical history of habitual cough includes a dry, chronic cough characterized by a honking sound and is present throughout the day, but absent at nighttime.[29] Although this entity may follow an upper respiratory illness, it is defined as separate from neurogenic cough, the latter of which is believed to be more strictly a disorder of peripheral nerves and brainstem reflexes. Habitual cough remains a controversial entity, as there is no specific proof as to its existence. Despite this, it is important to consider this diagnosis in the evaluation and management of patients with persistent cough despite an otherwise negative workup. Cortical factors likely play a major role in behavioral approaches for the treatment of both neurogenic and psychogenic chronic cough. These behavioral interventions, which are thought to reduce symptoms of cough severity, include cough suppression therapy, speech therapy, mindfulness, meditation, suggestion therapy, biofeedback, and cognitive behavioral therapy.[30–32] However, exactly how these approaches interact with cognitive processes require future investigation.

What *is* currently known of cortical and subcortical influences can be extrapolated from animal studies using retrograde viruses to identify pathways involved in cough and upper airway hyperresponsiveness. Specifically, the sensorimotor cortex becomes active during sensations of increased resistive load, suggesting this area of the brain has direct influences on mechanical stimulation (mechanoreceptors) but not chemical stimulation (chemoreceptors). The insula and cingulate cortex may have more to do with affective processing than discriminative processing of severity of sensations. These two cortical areas are thought to play a role in the perception of unpleasantness of laryngeal irritants by attributing emotion and cognition to the sensory experience.[33] This area of the brain may also be where the urge to cough is activated. Future work focusing on these areas of the brain in the context of coughing behaviors should be further explored. Prospective studies comparing actual threshold responses and the effect of emotional influences on laryngeal hyperresponsiveness are also needed to determine the roles neurological, immunological, and psychological factors play in chronic cough.

NOVEL PHARMACOLOGICAL AND SURGICAL TREATMENT APPROACHES

Unlike traditional treatments aimed at symptom control, novel pharmacological and surgical approaches have been proposed to address the elusive intersections of motor and sensory neuropathies that underlie chronic cough symptomology. Neuromodulating agents such as gabapentin, amitriptyline, pregabalin, and baclofen have emerged as first-line treatments for chronic neurogenic cough, with variable but generally favorable results. These agents have been reviewed earlier in this text in Chapter 6, as well as in many systematic reviews in recent years.[34–37]

Tramadol

A single-patient report of efficacy in treating chronic cough with tramadol was published in 2009.[38] Recently, Dion et al published a prospective case series of 16 patients with neurogenic cough who were treated with 50 mg of tramadol every 8 hours as needed.[39] Symptoms were assessed using the validated Cough Severity Index (CSI) and Leicester Cough Questionnaire (LCQ) before and after treatment; subjects were included if questionnaires were completed after a minimum of 14 days of treatment. The authors found statistically significant improvement in mean scores following treatment with tramadol. Side effects were minimal, with the most common being somnolence, reported in four out of 16 subjects.[39]

Glottic Insufficiency and Chronic Cough

Insofar as glottic insufficiency has been proposed as a possible underlying etiology for chronic cough, there have been investigations into the role of vocal fold augmentation to treat chronic cough. Vocal fold augmentation is designed to improve glottal closure through the use of an injectable implant (or filler) or through medialization laryngoplasty (surgical placement of a solid implant within the substance of the vocal folds). Injection augmentation can be performed in the operating room under general anesthesia but is frequently performed in the office setting under local anesthesia. The procedure involves inserting a needle into the vocal folds and using one of several available augmentation fillers. Multiple techniques have been described,[40–42] with the goal being to allow the vocal folds to be in full contact during the glottal cycle. Figure 10–1 shows an image before and after injection augmentation.

Crawley et al first described the use of injection augmentation to treat chronic cough in 2015 in a case series of six patients, five of whom reported improvement in CSI scores following injection laryngoplasty to address a diagnosis of chronic cough coupled with vocal fold paresis.[43] More recently,

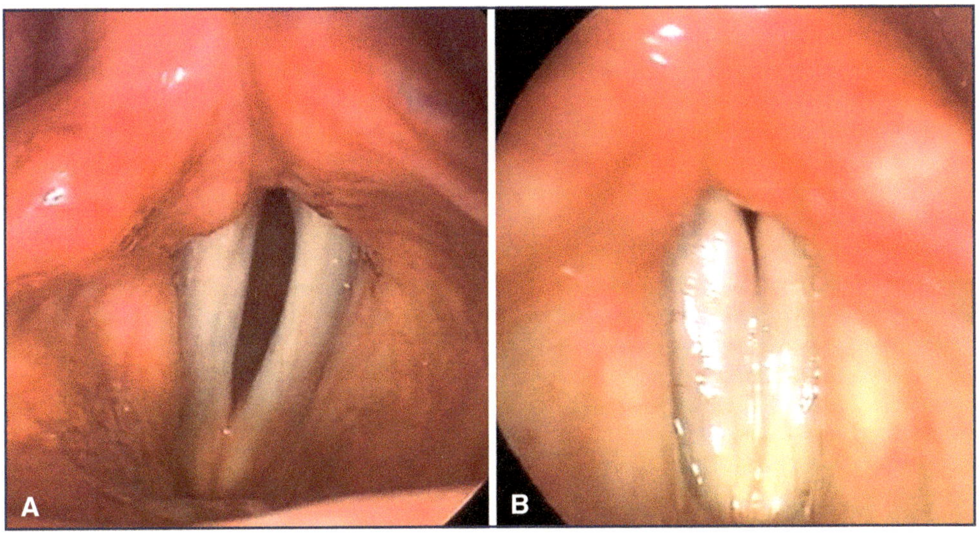

Figure 10–1. A. Preaugmentation. **B.** Postaugmentation.

Litts et al published a retrospective case series of 23 patients, most of whom (21 out of 23) presented with vocal fold atrophy as the etiology of their glottic insufficiency; the other two had sulcus vocalis or unilateral vocal fold paresis. Fourteen out of the 23 patients underwent behavioral therapy to reduce symptoms. Twenty-one out of the 23 underwent augmentation with Radiesse voice gel, and the remaining two underwent augmentation with Restylane. Nineteen underwent augmentation in the office; the remaining four underwent the procedure in the operating room. Eighteen of 23 patients underwent bilateral augmentation. The CSI was administered before and after treatment. The authors noted a significant reduction in the mean CSI score following injection laryngoplasty. Furthermore, they noted that 11 patients reported a return of symptoms at the 4-month post-injection visit, when the material was thought to have resorbed; eight of these patients went on to proceed with a permanent laryngoplastic procedure.[44]

Botox

Botulinum toxin has also been used in an effort to treat chronic cough through injections into the thyroarytenoid muscle. Sipp and colleagues produced one of the earliest reports of Botox injections into the thyroarytenoid muscles in three children with refractory habit cough. The authors described injection of 5 units of botulinum toxin A into each thyroarytenoid muscle under direct laryngoscopy; in each of the three patients, this resulted in cessation of the habit cough, though in one patient the cough resolved immediately following the procedure, well before Botox is known to peak in effect.[45]

Chu and colleagues described the use of Botox to treat chronic cough in a small case series of four adults. In this series, all patients were reported to have complete resolution of cough after a median of seven injections into the bilateral thyroarytenoid muscles with a mean dose of 4.0 units.[46] Subsequently, Sasieta et al published a retrospective case series of 22 patients with chronic cough treated with bilateral Botox-A injections. Treatment success was measured as 50% or greater subjective improvement in cough during a scripted phone call, 2 months after a Botox treatment session. The authors reported that 11 out of the 22 patients (50%) self-reported improvement of 50% or more of cough severity symptoms. Minor complications of transient postprocedural liquid dysphagia and dysphonia were also reported.[47]

Superior Laryngeal Nerve Block

Efforts to blunt the hypersensitivity of the larynx and to modulate the neurologic feedback loop have further manifested recently in a novel procedure to locally anesthetize the territory of the superior laryngeal nerve (SLN) with a field block. Simpson and colleagues described this procedure in a recent retrospective chart review of 18 patients who underwent SLN nerve block for treatment of chronic cough. The procedure involved an injection of a 50:50 solution of a long-acting particulate steroid and a local anesthetic, delivered via a 27-gauge needle at the entry point of the internal branch of the SLN in the posterior thyrohyoid membrane. Thirteen of the 18 patients included underwent unilateral injections, and five underwent bilateral injections; of the unilateral injections, 10 were left-sided. The patients underwent a mean of 2.4 SLN block procedures, with mean follow-up time following injection of 85.4 days. Outcomes were measured with pre- and posttreatment CSI scores; these scores decreased significantly from mean 26.8 pretreatment to 14.6 posttreatment.[48]

THINKING OUTSIDE OF THE BOX

Chronic cough as a clinical entity has been acknowledged for more than a century, yet underlying mechanisms are still not well understood. However, the variety of clinical presentations and trigger types suggest mechanisms are likely heterogeneous. Various clinical presentations have been attributed to chronic cough: hoarseness, dyspnea, and globus sensation, to name a few. It is unclear whether these symptoms should be lumped into chronic cough symptomology, whether they fall on a continuum, or whether they reflect common co-occurring yet distinct pathology, such as asthma, paradoxical vocal fold motion disorder (PVFM), and muscle tension dysphonia. Unfortunately, because of the overlap in clinical presentations between chronic cough and other laryngeal- or pulmonary-based pathology, and due to poor understanding of underlying mechanisms driving these clinical expressions, these entities are often lumped together under the same umbrella terms and nomenclature (eg, Irritable Larynx Syndrome). The downside to this approach is that just because symptoms overlap does not mean the underlying mechanisms driving these clinical expressions are the same. Therefore, more focus on the typical role of the larynx and the mechanisms causing dysfunction may be a beneficial approach to guide future investigations and clinical care than grouping these pathologies based on symptoms or triggers.

Various roles of the larynx can be divided into three concepts: airway protection (gatekeeping), ventilatory modulation (respiratory conduit), and communication. Underlying mechanisms involved in these laryngeal tasks are a part of various physiological, neurological, and biomechanical holarchical systems. These systems represent a relationship between entities that are part of a unique identity, but are also made up of subparts and are themselves subparts of a larger whole. The concept of holarchy is different from hierarchy in that the relationships can go "up and down" as well as "side to side." Conceptually, this can be thought of as multiple sets of nesting dolls with interchangeable parts. For instance, neurological pathways for coughing and breathing both travel and overlap in the nucleus ambiguus in the medulla. However, discharge patterns within the brainstem will rearrange based on upstream cortical input, which leads to distinct laryngeal behaviors, such as coughing and breathing, despite their neurophysiological and structural overlap in the brainstem.[2] This may be why patients with spasmodic dysphonia, a local laryngeal dystonia, are able to cough, laugh, and cry, but are unable to use the same laryngeal mechanism for speech.[49]

When the larynx takes on the role of gatekeeper, it does so to protect the lower respiratory tract. Therefore, it is probably no coincidence the true vocal folds are shelflike, with "down-turned free margins" functioning as a one-way valve.[50] The larynx is also smaller in diameter than the trachea and other sublaryngeal structures, which prevents larger particulate matter from entering the conducting airways, although this method of protection is not foolproof, and anything that can get past the larynx inevitably ends up in the (frequently right) bronchi.[50,51] This laryngeal gatekeeping can present as various glottal reflexes (ie, cough, aspiration, swallowing, apneic, and expiratory reflexes), which all involve some combination of vocal fold constriction and a period of apnea.[23,52–55]

Specific to cough, the cough reflex is a vagal response to irritants, influenced by chemoreceptors in the supraglottic or glottic region. This reflex prevents inhaled foreign particulates from entering the gas-exchanging area of the lungs. Cough is characterized by a sharp inspiratory phase, a compressive phase, and a short, ballistic expulsive phase.[56–59] During a reflexive cough, the true vocal folds, aryepiglottic folds, and oblique/transverse arytenoids act as one to create a single, continuous sphincter, completely closing the laryngeal inlet.[60] When the glottis is compressed, intrathoracic pressures increase to 250 to 300 mm Hg. While the abdomen contracts, the glottis opens abruptly to expel about 12 L/s of air (and hopefully the foreign particulate matter with it) through the vocal tract. The intrinsic laryngeal muscle adductors (lateral cricoarytenoids, interarytenoids, and thyroarytenoids) create glottal pressure while the posterior cricoarytenoids (and possibly cricothyroid) activate(s) to quickly abduct the vocal folds for airway clearance. Intercostal and abdominal respiratory muscles contract in conjunction with the glottis during both glottal closure and the expulsive phase.[2] When the system becomes hyperreactive or hyperresponsive, these patterns can come in the form of chronic cough or laryngospasm.

In contrast, when the larynx takes on the role of respiratory conduit for ventilatory needs, it tightly couples with the pulmonary musculature to maintain appropriate levels of intrathoracic and intrapulmonary pressure from one cyclical respiratory phase to the next. This is different from the short ballistic patterns involved in cough and other modes of airway protection (eg, deglutition). In respiratory roles, the larynx only closes partially during respiratory tasks to create appropriate levels of subglottal and transglottal pressures as well as intrapulmonary pressures.[2,61] Supralaryngeal structures also help maintain appropriate inspiratory pressures; however, with too much pressure, breathing can become disordered. For example, stenotic nostrils, especially when coupled with an elongated velum, have been shown to produce excessive negative inspiratory pressure above the laryngeal inlet, resulting in eversion of the laryngeal ventricles. This pressure "literally suck[s] the soft ventricular tissue out of its recess and into the laryngeal lumen," causing stridor and respiratory distress.[50]

These respiratory laryngeal patterns also become important for different bioenergetic and energy metabolism needs. For example, during prolonged or vigorous activity, respiratory drive increases, and the larynx works in conjunction with the pulmonary system to decrease pulmonary musculature workload and increase ventilatory capability to meet the metabolic needs of the system across respiratory cycles. To accomplish this task, the cross-sectional diameter of the lumen within the larynx increases by way of the arytenoids.[50] When discoordination occurs between the upper and lower respiratory tracts, this can result in aberrant vocal fold patterns from one respiratory cycle to the next. One example of these aberrant clinical patterns, commonly referred to as exercise-induced paradoxical vocal fold motion disorder (E-PVFM), involves the vocal folds' adduction toward the midline, paradoxical of metabolic needs.

Physiological differences between various roles of the larynx for airway protection and ventilation highlight the importance of treating corollary dysfunctions as separate entities (eg, chronic cough and PVFM, respectively). In the former, pulmonary and laryngeal patterns involve acute ballistic neuromuscular activation that results in acute apneic events (ie, cough). In fact, the task of cough temporarily overrides ventilatory needs to protect the airways. In the latter, patterns involve temporal cyclical respiratory dyscoordination leading to dyspnea. Mechanistic differences in physiological patterns and metabolic needs suggest chronic cough and PVFM—at least certain trigger variants like exertion-induced PVFM—are likely discrete entities and should be treated as such when creating study designs in future investigations and planning course of treatment in clinical settings.

Figure 10–2 is a visual representation of a proposed analytical framework to systematically evaluate mechanisms involved in laryngeal behaviors and resultant pathological symptoms. The schematic is

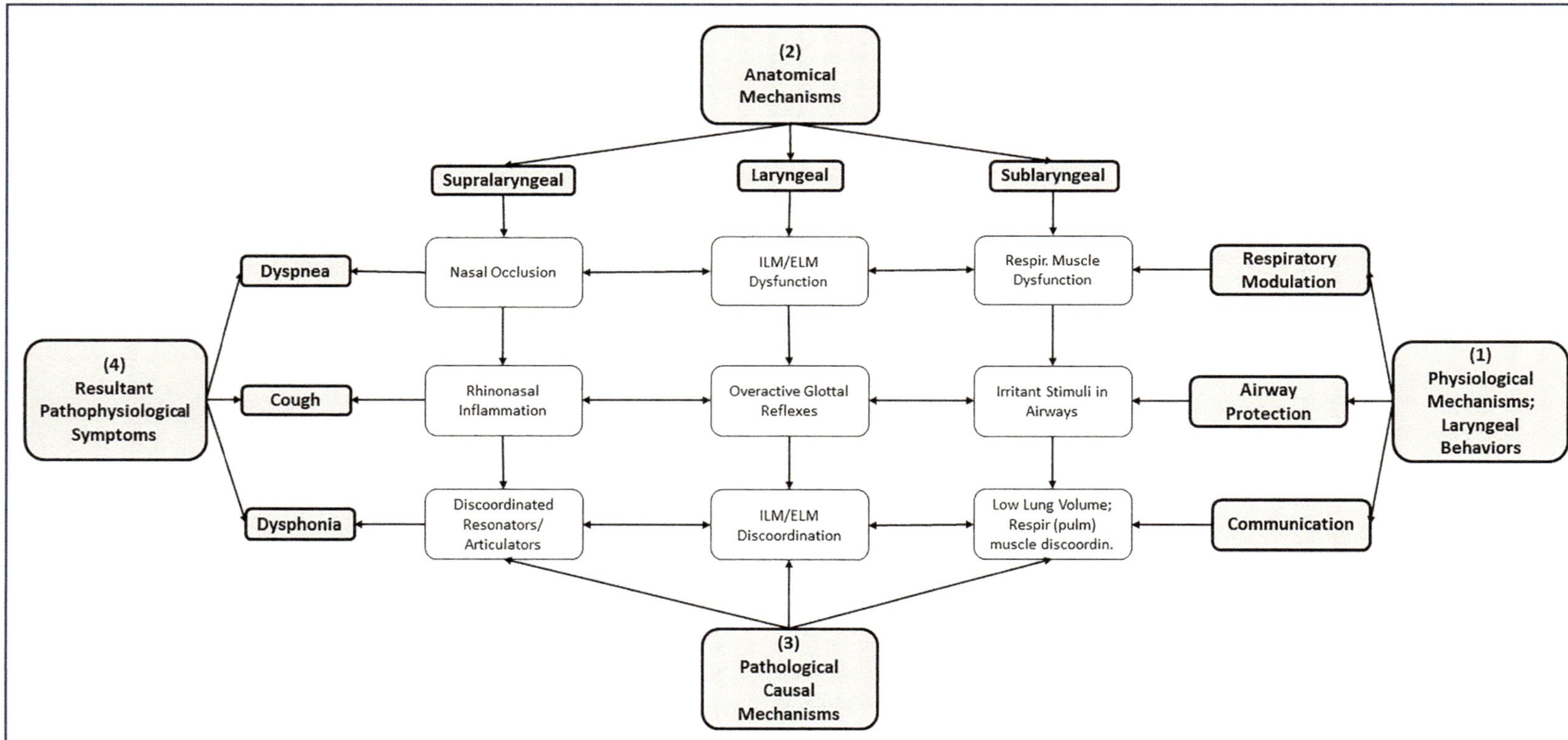

Figure 10–2. Physiological and pathophysiological mechanisms involved in various laryngeal behaviors including cough-, dyspneic-, and other laryngeal-related pathology (ILM = intrinsic laryngeal muscles; ELM = extrinsic laryngeal muscles).

by no means comprehensive; the goal is to illustrate the benefit of treating pathology related to the larynx (eg, chronic cough and PVFM) as separate entities. This approach can involve the study of normal physiological mechanisms involved in laryngeal behaviors (respiratory modulation, airway protection, and communication); the influences of structural or anatomical origin (at the supralaryngeal, laryngeal, and sublaryngeal levels); examples of pathological causal mechanisms (white boxes); and resultant pathophysiological symptoms (eg, dyspnea, cough, dysphonia).

TAKE HOME POINTS

- Recent efforts to address chronic cough highlight the multidisciplinary approach likely to bring clinicians and scientists across the next frontiers in the diagnosis, treatment, and management of chronic cough.
- Novel treatments for chronic cough include lidocaine blocks of the superior laryngeal nerve, botulinum toxin injection to the intrinsic laryngeal muscles, injection augmentation in cases of cough with glottis insufficiency, and neuromodulating medications.
- Translational and clinical investigations will be equally important in elucidating both biochemical and pathophysiological mechanisms and pathways, as well as applying these discoveries to meaningful and durable treatments to more definitively resolve symptoms.
- One of the fundamental quandaries in tackling chronic cough is the multiple contributing etiologies to the disease process, from the cellular level to the multiorgan interactions of human respirations; this should remind all who read and write on this topic that the way forward is best found in collaboration across disciplines and domains.

REFERENCES

1. Bolser DC, Davenport PW. Functional organization of the central cough generation mechanism. *Pulm Pharmacol Ther.* 2002;15(3):221–225.
2. Bolser DC, Poliacek I, Jakus J, Fuller DD, Davenport PW. Neurogenesis of cough, other airway defensive behaviors and breathing: a holarchical system? *Respir Physiol Neurobiol.* 2006;152(3):255–265.

3. Boushey HA, Richardson PS, Widdicombe JG. Reflex effects of laryngeal irritation on the pattern of breathing and total lung resistance. *J Physiol.* 1972;(2): 501–513.
4. Cobeta I, Pacheco A, Mora E. The role of the larynx in chronic cough. *Acta Otorrinolaringol Esp.* 2013;64(5):363–368. doi:10.1016/j.otorri.2012.10.001
5. Fontana GA, Lavorini F. Cough motor mechanisms. *Respir Physiol Neurobiol.* 2006;152(3):266–281.
6. Irwin RS, Curley FJ, French CL. Chronic cough: the spectrum and frequency of causes, key components of the diagnostic evaluation, and outcome of specific therapy. *Am Rev Respir Dis.* 1990;141(3):640–647.
7. Rolla G, Colagrande P, Magnano M, et al. Extrathoracic airway dysfunction in cough associated with gastroesophageal reflux. *J Allergy Clin Immunol.* 1998; 102(2):204–209.
8. Vertigan AE, Bone SL, Gibson PG. Laryngeal sensory dysfunction in laryngeal hypersensitivity syndrome. *Respirology.* 2013;18(6):948–956. doi:10.1111/resp.12103
9. Widdicombe JG. Afferent receptors in the airways and cough. *Respir Physiol.* 1998;114(1):5–15.
10. Chung KF. Chronic "cough hypersensitivity syndrome": a more precise label for chronic cough. *Pulm Pharmacol Ther.* 2011;24(3);267–271.
11. Milgrom H, Corsello P, Freedman M, Blager FB, Wood RP. Differential diagnosis and management of chronic cough. *Compr Ther.* 1990;16(10);46–53.
12. Dicpinigaitis PV, Lim L, Farmakidis C. Cough syncope. *Respir Med.* 2014;108(2): 244–251. doi:10.1016/j.rmed.2013.10.020
13. Minassian VA, Drutz HP, Al-Badr A. Urinary incontinence as a worldwide problem. *Int J Gynaecol Obstet.* 2003;82(3):327–338. doi:10.1016/S0020-7292(03)00220-0
14. Puetz TR, Vakil N. Gastroesophageal reflux-induced cough syncope. *Am J Gastroenterol.* 1995;90(12):2204–2206.
15. Morrison M, Rammage L, Emami AJ. The irritable larynx syndrome. *J Voice.* 1999;13(3):447–455.
16. Taramarcaz P, Grissell TV, Borgas T, Gibson PG. Transient postviral vocal cord dysfunction. *J Allergy Clin Immunol.* 2004;114(6):1471.
17. Ayres JG, Mansur AH. Vocal cord dysfunction and severe asthma: considering the total airway. *Am J Respir Crit Care Med.* 2011;184(1):2–3.
18. Chandra RK, Gerber ME, Holinger LD. Histological insight into the pathogenesis of severe laryngomalacia. *Int J Pediatr Otorhinolaryngol.* 2001;61(1):31–38.
19. Orenstein SR. An overview of reflux-associated disorders in infants: apnea, laryngospasm, and aspiration. *Am J Med.* 2001;111(8):60–63.
20. Thach MD, Bradley T. Reflux associated apnea in infants: evidence for a laryngeal chemoreflex. *Am J Med.* 1997;103(5):120S–124S.
21. Barnes PJ. Neurogenic inflammation in the airways. *Respir Physiol.* 2001;125(1): 145–154.
22. Weigand LA, Undem BJ. Allergen-induced neuromodulation in the respiratory tract. http://www.karger.com/Article/Abstract/336508. Published 2012. Accessed October 7, 2014.
23. Couto M, de Diego A, Perpiñi M, Delgado L, Moreira A. Cough reflex testing with inhaled capsaicin and TRPV1 activation in asthma and comorbid conditions. *J Investig Allergol Clin Immunol.* 2013;23(5):289–301.

24. Morris MJ, Deal LE, Bean DR, Grbach VX, Morgan JA. Vocal cord dysfunction in patients with exertional dyspnea. *Chest.* 1999;116(6):1676–1682.
25. Gimenez LM, Zafra H. Vocal cord dysfunction: an update. *Ann Allergy Asthma Immunol.* 2011;106(4):267–274.
26. Ibrahim WH, Gheriani HA, Almohamed AA, Raza T. Paradoxical vocal cord motion disorder: past, present and future. *Postgrad Med J.* 2007;83(977):164–172.
27. Reidenbach MM. Aryepiglottic fold: normal topography and clinical implications. *Clin Anat.* 1998;11(4):223–235.
28. Van den Bergh O, Van Diest I, Dupont L, Davenport PW. On the psychology of cough. *Lung.* 2012;190(1):55–61.
29. Haydour Q, Alahdab F, Farah M, et al. Management and diagnosis of psychogenic cough, habit cough, and tic cough: a systematic review. *Chest.* 2014;146(2): 355–372.
30. Young EC, Brammer C, Owen E, et al. The effect of mindfulness meditation on cough reflex sensitivity. *Thorax.* 2009;64(11):993–998. doi:10.1136/thx.2009.116723
31. Labbé EE. Biofeedback and cognitive coping in the treatment of pediatric habit cough. *Appl Psychophysiol Biofeedback.* 2006;31(2):167–172. doi:10.1007/s10484-006-9007-5
32. Powell C, Brazier A. Psychological approaches to the management of respiratory symptoms in children and adolescents. *Paediatr Respir Rev.* 2004;5(3):214–224. doi:10.1016/j.prrv.2004.04.010
33. Davenport PW, Vovk A. Cortical and subcortical central neural pathways in respiratory sensations. *Respir Physiol Neurobiol.* 2009;167(1):72–86.
34. Giliberto JP, Cohen SM, Misono S. Are neuromodulating medications effective for the treatment of chronic neurogenic cough? *Laryngoscope.* 2017;127(5):1007.
35. Cohen SM, Misono S. Use of specific neuromodulators in the treatment of chronic, idiopathic cough: a systematic review. *Otolaryngol Head Neck Surg.* 2013;148(3):374–382.
36. Dicpinigaitis PV. Current and future peripherally-acting antitussives. *Respir Physiol Neurobiol.* 2006;152(3):356–362.
37. Gibson PG, Vertigan AE. Speech pathology for chronic cough: a new approach. *Pulm Pharmacol Ther.* 2009;22(2):159–162.
38. Louly PG, Medeiros-Souza P, Santos-Neto L. N-of-1 double-blind, randomized controlled trial of tramadol to treat chronic cough. *Clin Ther.* 2009;31(5):1007–1013.
39. Dion GR, Teng SE, Achlatis E, Fang Y, Amin MR. Treatment of neurogenic cough with tramadol: a pilot study. *Otolaryngol Head Neck Surg.* 2017;157(1):77–79.
40. Mallur PS, Rosen CA. Vocal fold injection: review of indications, techniques, and materials for augmentation. *Clin Exp Otorhinolaryngol.* 2010;3(4):177.
41. Sulica L, Rosen CA, Postma GN, et al. Current practice in injection augmentation of the vocal folds: indications, treatment principles, techniques, and complications. *Laryngoscope.* 2010;120(2):319–325.
42. Amin MR. Thyrohyoid approach for vocal fold augmentation. *Ann Otol Rhinol Laryngol.* 2006;115(9):699–702.
43. Crawley BK, Murry T, Sulica L. Injection augmentation for chronic cough. *J Voice.* 2015;29(6):763–767.
44. Litts JK, Fink DS, Clary MS. The effect of vocal fold augmentation on cough symptoms in the presence of glottic insufficiency. *Laryngoscope.* 2018;128(6): 1316–1319.

45. Sipp JA, Haver KE, Masek BJ, Hartnick CJ. Botulinum toxin A: a novel adjunct treatment for debilitating habit cough in children. *Ear Nose Throat J.* 2007;86(9): 570–572.
46. Chu MW, Lieser JD, Sinacori JT. Use of botulinum toxin type A for chronic cough: a neuropathic model. *Arch Otolaryngol Head Neck Surg.* 2010;136(5):447–452.
47. Sasieta HC, Iyer VN, Orbelo DM, et al. Bilateral thyroarytenoid botulinum toxin type A injection for the treatment of refractory chronic cough. *JAMA Otolaryngol Head Neck Surg.* 2016;142(9):881–888.
48. Simpson CB, Tibbetts KM, Loochtan MJ, Dominguez LM. Treatment of chronic neurogenic cough with in-office superior laryngeal nerve block. *Laryngoscope.* 2018;128(8):1898–1903.
49. Ludlow CL. Central nervous system control of the laryngeal muscles in humans. *Respir Physiol Neurobiol.* 2015;147(2):205–222.
50. Kirchner JA. The vertebrate larynx: adaptations and aberrations. *Laryngoscope.* 1993;103(10):1197–1201.
51. Brooks S. Anatomy of the cough reflex. *Cough.* 2011;7(10):1–26.
52. Eccles R. Upper airway reflexes and involvement of the lower airway. *Lung Biol Health Dis.* 2003;181:87–99.
53. Murakami Y, Kirchner JA. Respiratory movements of the vocal cords. An electromyographic study in the cat. *Laryngoscope.* 1972;82(3):454–467.
54. Murakami Y, Kirchner JA. Mechanical and physiological properties of reflex laryngeal closure. *Ann Otol Rhinol Laryngol.* 1972;81(1):59.
55. Widdicombe J. Respiratory reflexes. In: Holgate ST, Koren HS, Samet JM, Maynard RL, eds. *Air Pollution and Health.* London, UK: Elsevier; 1999:325–340.
56. Butani L, O'Connell EJ. Functional respiratory disorders. *Ann Allergy Asthma Immunol.* 1997;79(2):91–101.
57. Hoyte FC. Vocal cord dysfunction. *Immunol Allergy Clin North Am.* 2013;33(1): 1–22.
58. Kenn K, Balkissoon R. Vocal cord dysfunction: what do we know? *Eur Respir J.* 2011;37(1):194–200. doi:10.1183/09031936.00192809
59. Sasaki MDCT, Weaver MDEM. Physiology of the larynx. *Am J Med.* 1997;103(5): 9S–18S.
60. Lumb AB. Functional anatomy of the respiratory tract. In: *Nunn's Applied Respiratory Physiology.* 7th ed. London, UK: Elsevier; 2010:13–26.
61. Gautier H, Remmers JE, Bartlett D. Control of the duration of expiration. *Respir Physiol*, 1973;18(2):205–221.

INDEX

Note: Page numbers in **bold** reference non-text subjects.

A

Abdominal
- fat, reflux and, 71
- glottal reflex responses, 188–189
- motility, TNE and, 129

ACCP (American College of Chest Physicians), 49
- cough guidelines, 49, 51
- Cough-Specific Quality-of-Life Questionnaire (CQLQ), 11
- evidence-based guidelines updated, 45
- UACS (Upper airway cough syndrome) introduced by, 49
  - defined by, 7

ACE (Angiotensin converting enzyme) inhibitors, 68, 180
- chronic cough and, 8–9, 45
- cough and, 49, 187
- GERD and, 66–67

Achalasia, dysplasia and, 134

Acid
- esophageal-tracheobronchial cough reflex and, 67
- suppression, 175
- taste in mouth, GERD and, 66

ACOS (Asthma-chronic obstructive pulmonary disease overlap syndrome), 22

Activities of daily living (ADL), 13

Acute
- adenoid hypertrophy, 49
- asthma, Dead Sea salt and, 54
- bronchoconstriction, SABAs and, 28
- cough, defined, 10.16
- upper respiratory infection, inhaled anticholinergics and, 53

Adenoiditis, 49

ADL (Activities of daily living), 13

AERD (Aspirin-exacerbated respiratory disease), 22

Aeroallergen piolysensitization, EoE and, 133

Aerodigestive tract, aspiration and, 67

Afferent nerves, 188

Afrin, 127

Age, dysphagia and, 134–135

Airflow obstruction, variability in measurement of, 24–26

Airway
- convergence of, afferent sensations and, 99
- edema, 22
  - stretch receptors and, 3
- eosinophilia, 22
- foreign bodies, 132
- hyperresponsiveness, 22
- inflammation, 22
  - in asthma, 42
- mucosal eosinophilia, 27
- obstruction, acute, 22
- salt concentration, Xylitol and, 53
- sensory nerves, 3

Albuterol, 28

Alcohol
- use of, physical examination and, 9
- vocal hygiene and, 147

Alginate therapy, 181

Alginates, 72

Allergens, 22
- bronchoconstriction and, 22
- cough reflex and, 46
- environmental, asthma and, 23
- nasal stimulus with, 44

Allergic
- salute, 10
- shiners, 10

Allergic rhinitis (AR), 40
- asthma and, 41

Allergic rhinitis (AR) *(continued)*
 described, 46
 intranasal hypertonic saline and, 54
 management of, 49
 saline irrigations and, 53
Alpha-delta afferents, 4
Alveolar carbon dioxide concentration ($PACO_2$), 162
Alveolar phospholipids, 83
American Academy of Otolaryngology--Head and Surgery, 86
American Bronchoesophagological Association, 86
American Cancer Society, recommends LDCT, 11
American College of Chest Physicians (ACCP)
 cough guidelines, 49, 51
 Cough-Specific Quality-of-Life Questionnaire (CQLQ), 11
 evidence-based guidelines updated, 45
 UACS (Upper airway cough syndrome) introduced by, 49
  defined by, 7
American College of Chest Physicians, UACS definition of, 7
American Gastroenterological Association, 86
American Geriatric Society, on amitriptyline, 106
American Medical Association, 159
American Society of Clinical Hypnosis (ASCH), 159
American Speech-Language-Hearing Association (ASHA), dysplasia defined, 119
American Speech-Language Hearing Association, 147
American Thoracic Society, 32
Amitriptyline, 104–106, 190
Amyloidosis., 69
 sarcoidosis and, 10
Andidiasis, TNE and, 129
Anesthesia
 FEES and, 127
 LEMG and, 103
Angiotensin receptor blockers, cough and, 68
Angiotensin-converting-enzyme (ACE) inhibitors, 68, 180
 chronic cough and, 8–9
 cough and, 49, 187
 GERD and, 66–67
Anterior ethmoid disease, 48–49
Antibiofilm properties, Xylitol and, 53
Anticholinergic effects, of amitriptyline, 106
Antigen inflammation, neuropeptides and, 99
Antimicrobial activity, Xylitol and, 53
Antireflux surgery, 73–74, 182
 chronic cough and, 175
 efficacy of, 86–87
 refractory chronic cough and, 182
Anxiety, chronic cough and, 13
Apneas, 188
AR (Allergic rhinitis), 40
 asthma and, 41
 described, 46
 intranasal hypertonic saline and, 54
 management of, 49
 saline irrigations and, 53
ASCH (American Society of Clinical Hypnosis), 159
ASHA (American Speech- Language-Hearing Association), dysplasia defined, 119
Aspiration, 82
 achalasia and, 134
 chronic cough and, 117
 defined, 126
 foreign bodies, 132
 oropharyngeal dysphagia and, 118
 pneumonia, 117
  dysplasia and, 118
 predicting risk of, 119
 of sinonasal drainage, 45
Aspirin
 asthma and, 23
 reflux and, 72
Aspirin-exacerbated respiratory disease (AERD), 22
Asthma, 5, 40
 airway inflammation in, 42

chronic rhinosinusitis (CRS) and, clinical relationship between, 43–44
cough and, 39, 49
cough-variant, 5, 21–35
diagnosis of, 23–24
hypersensitive cough reflex and, 22
manifests of, 21
treatment of, 28–33
Dead Sea salt and, 54
diagnosis of, 23–27
spirometry, 24
eosinophilic, 5
expiratory wheezing and, 10
manifestations of, 23
nonallergic rhinitis and, 42–45
clinical relationship between, 42–43
persistent, childhood asthma and, 23
refractory chronic cough and, 183
rhinitis and, 41
allergic, 41
theory of systemic amplification and, 45
tobacco and, 9
treatment of, 28–33
controller agents, 29–30
inhaled corticosteroids, 30–31
quick-relief bronchodilators, 28–29
Asthma-chronic obstructive pulmonary disease overlap syndrome (ACOS), 22
Atopic
asthma, 22
cough, 49
EoE and, 133
Attention, chronic cough and, 13
Autoimmune disease, dysplasia and, 135
Autonomic nervous system, vasomotor rhinitis and, 47

B

Baby shampoo, 54
Baclofen, 190
Bacteria, refluxate and, 65
BAL (Bronchoalveolar lavage), pepsin in, 82–84
Barium swallow (MBS), 125–126
Barrett's esophagus, TNE and, 129, 130
Basal intra-abdominal pressure, reflux and, 71
Bed, elevating head, reflux and, 72
Beta-blockers
bronchoconstriction and, 22
chronic cough and, 8
BHT (Breath-holding time), 162
Bile
acids, cell membrane blebbing and, 87
salts, refluxate and, 65
Biofeedback, 190
Biologic therapy, 30, 32–33
Biomarkers
in chronic cough, 81–84
in reflux, 81–84
Blebbing, cell membranes, 87
Block, superior laryngeal nerve, 192–193
Bogus tickle, 99
Bohr effect, 163
Boluses
administration of, 125–126
predicting aspiration risk with, 119
Botox injections, 182, 192
Botulinum toxin, injections, 182, 192
Brainstem, 99
Bravo reflux testing system, 70
BRAVO™ Reflux Testing System, 178
Breath
biomarker, exhaled, 27
shortness of, cough-variant asthma, 21
Breath-holding time (BHT), 162
Breathing
dysfunctional, Buteyko breathing method and, 160–164
nasal to mouth, 45
pattern, SLPs observation of, 151–152
relaxed throat, 156
Broken ribs, cough and, 2
Bronchial
hyperresponsiveness, 40
thermoplasty, 32–33, 182–183

Bronchiectasis, 68
Bronchitis
chronic, 68
eosinophilic, 5, 33, 49
Bronchoalveolar lavage (BAL), pepsin in, 82–84
Bronchoconstriction, 22
acute, SABAs and, 28
bronchoprovocation testing and, 22
exercise induced, 22
Bronchoconstrictor response, positive, and cold air, 44
Bronchodilators
quick-relief, 28–29
reversibility, 24–26
Bronchoprotective effect, tachyphylaxis to, 28
Bronchoprovocation, testing, 24–26, 181
Budesonide
intranasal, 43
pregnancy and, 48
Burns, Manuka honey and, 53–54
Buteyko, Konstantin, 163
Buteyko breathing method, 160–164, 181
retraining, 163–164

C

Caffeine
reflux and, 72
vocal hygiene and, 147
Calcium channel blockers, reflux and, 72
Cancer, chest roentgenogram and, 10
Capnography, end-tidal, 162
Capsaicin, 9, 54–55, 189
induced cough, 144
neurogenic cough and, 99
Carbonated beverages, reflux and, 72
Carcinoma, TNE and, 129
CAT (Computerized tomography), paranasal sinus and, 11
Caudal brainstem, central cough generator and, 4
Cell membranes, blebbing, 87
Central cough generator, 4
C-fibers, 4
Chart review, 122
Chemical
irritants
neurogenic cough and, 99
rhinitis and, 47–48
receptors, 3–4
Chemoreceptors, 4, **4**
Chest, 66–67
Chest
pain, retrosternal, GERD and, 66
roentgenogram, 10
tightness
asthma, childhood, 23
cough-variant asthma, 21
Childhood, asthma and, 23
Chili peppers, 54
Chocolate, reflux and, 72
Choking
GERD and, 66
patient referral and, 120–121
Cholinergic reflex, 44
Chronic
autoimmune disease, dysplasia and, 135
bronchitis, 7, 68
pain, neurogenic cough and, 99
Chronic cough, 188
ACE inhibitors and, 45
antireflux surgery and, 175
biomarkers in, 81–84
causes of, 4–8
asthma, 5
gastroesophageal reflux disease (GERD), 5–6
laryngopharyngeal reflux (LPR), 6
UCAS, 7
DB and, 160–164
defined, 1, 143
diagnosis of, 49–52
diet and, 71–72
dysphagia in, 117–137
dysphonia and, 145, 152
etiology of, 180
evaluation, 146–147
glottic insufficiency and, 191–192
hoarseness and, 179
idiopathic, 45

ILS and, 145
impact of, 11–14
economic, 12–13
quality of life, 13–14
lifestyles and, 71–72
LPR and, 65
medical history and, 51
medications, 8–9
middle ear effusion and, 180
multidisciplinary approach to, **14–15**
psychological factors associated with, 13
reflux and, 65
refractory, 14, 175, 183, 187
antireflux surgery and, 182
diagrammatic approach to, 178
LPR and, 175
SLPs and, 176
SLP management of, 144–145
smokers and, 9
as a symptom, 174
treatment algorithm, **177**
treatment of, 52–55, 159–164
hypnosis, 159–160
upper airway disorders linked to, 145–146
voice therapist and, 181
voice therapy and, 158
without evidence of PND, 46
see also Cough
Chronic obstructive pulmonary disease (COPD)
emphysema, and, 7
expiratory wheezing and, 10
management of, 49
Chronic rhinosinusitis (CRS), 41–42
asthma and, clinical relationship between, 43–44
GERD and, 44
laryngopharyngeal reflux (LPR) and, 44–45
management of, 49
Manuka honey and, 53–54
nasal polyps and, 41–42
saline irrigations and, 53
Xylitol and, 53
Cigarette smoke
asthma and, 23
cough and, 49
Citric acid, 54
Clinical swallow evaluation (CSE), 120–125, 121
bolus administration, 124–125
components of, 120–121
case history, 122
chart review, 121–122
indications of
client compliant, 122
symptoms history, 122–123
oral mechanism examination, 123–124
VFSS and, 125–126
Cobblestoning, of posterior pharyngeal mucosa, 46
Cognitive behavioral therapy, 190
Cold air
asthma and, 23
bronchoconstriction and, 22
lower airway resistance and, 44
positive bronchoconstrictor response and, 44
Colds, cough-variant asthma and, 23
Collapsed lung, cough and, 2
ComforTec LPR, probe array, 70
Comorbid pulmonary disease, 68
Computed tomography (CT), CRS and asthma correlation and, 43
Computerized tomography (CAT), paranasal sinus and, 11
Concentration, chronic cough and, 13
Concha bullosa, 48–49
Congestion
AR and, 46
venous, 9–10
Controller agents, 29–30
COPD (Chronic obstructive pulmonary disease)
emphysema, and, 7
expiratory wheezing and, 10
management of, 49
Cortical control, of cough, 4
Corticosteroids, inhaled, 30–31
Cottonoids, TNE and, 129
Cough
acute onset of, 100
asthma and, 5

Cough *(continued)*
capsaicin-induced, 144
central generator of, 4
chronic, 1
asthma and, 5
causes of, 4–8
chronic bronchitis, 7
GERD and, 5–6
LPR and, 6
UACS, 6–7
conscious suppression of, 4
constituents of, 2
control strategies, 155
defined, 2
dental pathology and, 49
described, 1, 187
diagnosis of, 49–52
habitual, 189
neurogenic *See* Neurogenic cough
neurophysiology of, 2–4
pathophysiology of, 2
patient referral and, 120–121
physiologic basis of, 2
psychogenic, 189
reflective pathways, 189–190
reflex sensitivity, 145
reflux related, surgery and, 73
reflux-related, 133–134
stimulated by reflux, 67
suppression/distracting techniques, 155–156
suppression therapy, 190
tic, 189
tobacco and, 9
treatment of, 52–55, 159–164
hypnosis, 159–160
upper respiratory tract infection (URTI) and, 144
see also Chronic cough
Cough reflex, 67
examination and, 118
hypersensitive, cough-variant asthma and, 22
hypersensitivity of, 47
laryngeal hypersensitivity syndromes and, 99
Cough Severity Index (CSI), 147, **148**, 191
Coughing, defined, 1, 7
Cough-Specific Quality-of-Life Questionnaire (CQLQ), 11
Cough-variant asthma, 5, 21–35, 49
childhood, 23
clinical manifestations of, 23
cough and, 68
diagnosis of, 23–27
spirometry, 24
variability in measurement flow and, 24–26
hypersensitive cough reflex and, 22
manifests of, 21
pathophysiology of, 21–22
treatment of, 28–33
biologic therapy, 32
bronchial thermoplasty, 32–33
controller agents, 29–30
inhaled corticosteroids, 30–31
LABAs, 31
leukotriene modifiers, 31–32
quick-relief bronchodilators, 28–29
CP (Cricopharyngeal) bar, 126
dysplasia and, 132
CQLQ (Cough-Specific Quality-of-Life Questionnaire), 11
Cricopharyngeal (CP) bar, 126
dysplasia and, 132
CRS (Chronic rhinosinusitis), 41–42
asthma and, clinical relationship between, 43–44
GERD and, 44
laryngopharyngeal reflux (LPR) and, 44–45
management of, 49
Manuka honey and, 53–54
nasal polyps and, 41–42
saline irrigations and, 53
theory of systemic amplification and, 45
Xylitol and, 53
CRSwNP, 41, 43
CSE (Clinical swallow evaluation), 120–125
bolus administration, 124–125
components of, chart review, 121–122

indications of, 120–121
client compliant, 122
symptoms history, 122–123
oral mechanism examination, 123–124
VFSS and, 125–126
CSI (Cough Severity Index), 147, **148**, 191
CT (Computer tomography), CRS and asthma correlation and, 43
Cytokines,
secretion of, 41
Th2, T-helper lymphocytes, 42, 43

D

Daytime fatigue, chronic cough and, 13
DB (Dysfunctional breathing)
Buteyko breathing method and, 160–164
diagnosis of, 162
prevalence of, 161–162
symptoms of, 161
Dead Sea salt, 54
Death, dysplasia and, 118
Dehydration, dysplasia and, 118
DeMeester score, 6, 70–71, **75**
Dental pathology, postnasal drainage/cough and, 49
Depression, chronic cough and, 13
Deviated nasal septum, 48
rhinitis and, 47
DI (Dyspnea Index), 147, **150**
Diagnostic tests, cost of, **12**
Diet, reflux and, 71–72
Digestive enzymes, refluxate and, 65
Distal chip digital laryngoscopy, visualization of larynx by, 102
Diuretics, chronic cough and, 8
Double pH probe, LPR and, 11
Dysfunctional breathing (DB)
Buteyko breathing method and, 160–164
diagnosis of, 162
prevalence of, 161–162
symptoms of, 161
Dysmotility, 180, 182
Dysphagia
achalasia and, 134
aging and, 134–135
in chronic cough, 117–137
clinical swallow examination, 120–125
CSE and, 120–125
defined, 119
EoE and, 133
FEES and, 127–128
food, vagal nerve dysfunction and, 100
foreign bodies and, 132
GERD and, 66
HRM and, 131
neurogenic cough and, 101
oropharyngeal, aspiration and, 118
PVV and, 82
reflux and, 133–134
screening, 118–120
TNE and, 128–130
vagal nerve dysfunction and, 100
VFSS and, 125–126
Zenker's diverticulum, 131–132
Dysphonia, 69
chronic cough and, 145, 152
laryngeal hypersensitivity syndromes and, 100
neurogenic cough and, 101
Dysplasia
autoimmune disease and, 135
eosinophilic esophagitis (EoE) and, 133
progressive systemic sclerosis and, 135
scleroderma and, 135
Dyspnea, 82
asthma and, 5
chronic cough and, 143
episodic, 145
Dyspnea Index (DI), 147, **150**
Dystonia, LPR and, 65

E

EAT-10 (Eating Assessment Tool), 119
Eating Assessment Tool (EAT-10), 119
Economic costs, chronic cough and, 12–13

Edema
airway, stretch receptors and, 3
subepithelial, 43
Efferent vagal motor response, 189
Efficacy of antireflux surgery, LPR, 86
Effusion, middle era, chronic cough and, 180
EGD (Esophagogastroduodenoscopy), 69
reflux and, 72
EGD (Gastroesophageal endoscopy), 175
EIB (Exercised-induced bronchoconstriction), 22
ELBDs (Episodic laryngeal breathing disorders), 145
Emotions
asthma and, 23
ILS and, 145
Emphysema,
described, 7
expiratory wheezing and, 10
tobacco and, 9
Endoscope, visualization of larynx with, 102
Endoscopic sinus surgery
CRS and, 44
saline irrigations and, 53
Endoscopy
laryngeal, 69
LPR and, 68–69
nasal, 52
Endosome marker Rab-9, 84
End-tidal
capnography, 162
carbon dioxide (ETCO2), 162
Environmental
allergens, asthma and, 23
irritants, rhinitis and, 47–48
EoE (Eosinophilic esophagitis), dysplasia and, 133
Eosinophile count, symptom scores and, 43
Eosinophilia
airway, 22
mucosal, airway, 27
Eosinophilic
asthma, 5
bronchitis, 5
cough and, 68
episodic choking, 82
mediated inflammation, 43
rhinosinusitis, 41
Eosinophilic esophagitis (EoE), dysplasia and, 133
Episodic chronic cough, acid exposure and, 67
Episodic laryngeal breathing disorders (ELBDs), 145
Epithelial damage, inflammation and, 43, 188
Esophageal
diverticula, TNE and, 129
dysmotility, vagal nerve dysfunction and, 100
sensory inputs, afferent sensations and, 99
sphincter, lower, TNE and, 129
tracheobronchial cough reflex, 67
Esophagitis
reflux, 69
TNE and, 129
Esophagogastroduodenoscopy (EGD)
Esophagopharyngeal reflux disease, HRM and, 131
Esophagus
esophageal-tracheobronchial cough reflex and, 67
jackhammer, 135
sensitivity to reflux, 86
TNE and, 129
Estill Voice Model, 156
$ETCO_2$ (End-tidal carbon dioxide), 162
European Community Respiratory Health Survey, 42
European Respiratory Society, 32
Exacerbation-prone asthma, 22
Exercise, asthma and, 23
Exercised-induced bronchoconstriction (EIB), 22
Expiratory wheezing, 10
Extraesophageal reflux disease, 87
Extrathoracic airway, vagal afferents and, **4**

F

Fatigue, chronic cough and, 13
Fecal incontinence, cough and, 2

Feeding intolerance, dysplasia and, 133
FEES (Flexible Endoscopic Evaluation of Swallowing), 127–128, 176
FEESST (Fiberoptic endoscopic evaluation of swallowing with sensory testing), 128
FHP (Forward head posture), breathing and, 156–157
Fiberoptic endoscopic evaluation of swallowing with sensory testing (FEESST), 128
Fiberoptic laryngoscope, visualization of larynx with, 10, 101
Fibrosis, subepithelial, 22
Flexible Endoscopic Evaluation of Swallowing (FEES), 127–128, 176
Flexible fiberoptic examination, gERD/LPR and, 10
Flexible fiberoptic laryngoscope, visualization of larynx with, 10, 101
Flexible laryngoscopy, 119
  visualization of larynx with, 102
Food
  allergens, EoE and, 133
  coming out nose, 121
  dysphagia, vagal nerve dysfunction and, 100
  impaction, 133
Foreign bodies, dysphagia and, 132
Forward head posture (FHP), breathing and, 156–157
Fractional exhaled nitric oxide (F_{ENO}), 27
Fumes, asthma and, 23
Functional measurements, by SLPs, 152–153
Fundoplication, 73, 76, 87
  laparoscopic, 86
  Nissen, 74, 83, 87, 182
Futicasone, pregnancy and, 48

G

GABA analogs, 106
Gabapentin, 104, 107–109, 190
Gastric
  bypass, 74, 76
  emptying, decreased, 182
  pepsin, refluxate and, 65
  reflux, 6
Gastroesophageal endoscopy (EGD), 175
Gastroesophageal reflux disease (GERD), 5–6, 39, 65
  chronic cough and, 46
  cough and, 49
  CRS and, 44
  described, 66
  diagnosis of, 175
  eosinophilic esophagitis and, 133
  ILS and, 98
  PPIs and, 86
  prevalence of, 66–67
  surgery and, 44, 73, 86
  vagal nerve dysfunction and, 100
Gastroesophageal reflux (GER)
  described, 65
  GERD and, 66
  ILS and, 145
Gaviscon Advance, 72, 181
GER (Gastroesophageal reflux)
  described, 65
  GERD and, 66
  ILS and, 145
GERD (Gastroesophageal reflux disease), 5–6, 39, 65
  chronic cough and, 46, 49
  CRS and, 44
  DeMeester score and, 6, 70–71, **75**
  described, 66
  diagnosis of, 175
  eosinophilic esophagitis and, 133
  ILS and, 98
  PPIs and, 86
  prevalence of, 66–67
  surgery and, 44, 73, 86
  vagal nerve dysfunction and, 100
GERD/LPR, **14**
  flexible fiberoptic examination and, 10
  pathophysiologic mechanism, 6
Globus
  chronic cough and, 143
  laryngeal hypersensitivity syndromes and, 100
  neurogenic cough and, 101

Globus *(continued)*
pharyngeus, 69, 145–146
GERD and, 6
ILS and, 145
sensation, 82
LPR and, 65
PVV and, 82
Glottal reflex responses, abnormal, 188–189
Glottic insufficiency, 69, 182
chronic cough and, 191–192
Glottis, amyloid in, 10
Glycosaminoglycan, 54
Goblet cell hyperplasia, 43
Granulomatosis with polyangitis (Wegener's) deposits, sarcoidosis and, 10

H

H2 blockers, 72
Habitual cough, 189
Halitosis, GERD and, 66
Haller cells, 48
Head
elevating, reflux and, 72
examination of, chronic cough and, 9
Heart
disease, tobacco and, 9
failure, expiratory wheezing and, 10
Heartburn
GERD and, 6
postprandial, GERD and, 66
surgery and, 73
vagal nerve dysfunction and, 100
Helicobacter pylori, 44
HEMII-pH, 86, 87, 170, 175–182
testing, 72
Herpes simplex virus, 47
Hiatal hernia
surgery and, 73
TNE and, 129–130
High-resolution esophageal manometry (HRM), 131, 176, 180
Histamine, 22
Hoarseness, chronic cough and, 179
Hopkins rod laryngoscopes, 102
Hormonal rhinitis, 47–48
HRM (High-resolution esophageal manometry), 131, 176, 180
HVS (Hyperventilation syndrome), 161
Hydrochloric acid
gastric reflux and, 6
refluxate and, 65
Hyperfunctional laryngeal symptoms, 98
Hyperplasia
goblet cell, 43
smooth muscle, 22
Hypersecretion, mucus, 43
Hypersensitive larynx syndrome, 192
neurogenic cough and, 100
Hypersensitivity, of cough reflex, 47
Hypertrophy, smooth muscle, 22
Hyperventilation, 162–163
Hyperventilation syndrome (HVS), 161
Hypnosis
cough treatment and, 159–160
defined, 159

I

Iatrogenic disease, 49
ICS (Inhaled corticosteroids), 30–31
Idiopathic chronic cough, 45
IL-5 (Interleukin-5), 41
Illness, preception, chronic cough and, 13
ILS (Irritable larynx syndrome)
laryngeal hyperfunction and, 98
neurogenic cough and, 100
Imaging, 10–11
Imaging scores, CT and, 43
Impedance/pH probes, 70
IMT (Inspiratory muscle strength training), 157
Indirect laryngoscopy, visualization of larynx with, 102
Infections
respiratory, bronchoconstriction and, 22
upper airway tract, asthma and, 23
Inferior turbinate hypertrophy, rhinitis and, 47
Inflammation
airway, 22
antigen/viral, neuropeptides and, 99

epithelial, 188
T-helper, 43
Inflammatory
diseases, pepsin as mediator of, 84–87
mediators, 158
Influenza virus, 47
Inhaled
allergens, bronchoconstriction and, 22
anticholinergics, 53
Inhaled corticosteroids (ICS), 30–31
Inhalers, steroid, 175
Injections
augmentation, 191
Botox, 182, 192
superior laryngeal nerve, 182
Inspiratory muscle strength training (IMT), 157
Interleukin-5 (IL-5), 41
Intracellular, damage, pepsin and, 6
Intranasal
budesonide, 43
corticosteroid spray, hormonal rhinitis and, 48
hypertonic saline, 54
Ipratropium, 53
bromide nasal spray, 53
Irrigations, saline, 53
Irritable larynx syndrome (ILS)
laryngeal hyperfunction and, 98
neurogenic cough and, 100
Irritants
bronchoconstriction and, 22
cough reflex and, 46
rhinitis and, 47

J

Jackhammer esophagus, 135
Jugular ganglia, 3

K

Killian's dehiscence, 131

L

LABAs (Long-acting beta agonists), 30, 31
Laparoscopic
antireflux surgery, 73
fundoplication, 86
Rou-en-Y gastric bypass, 74
LAR (Laryngeal adductor response), 128
Laryngeal
allergy, 69
deconstriction techniques, SLPs and, 156
dysesthesias, 98
electromyography (LEMG), 103
neurogenic cough and, 101
endoscopy, 69
hyperresponsiveness, 82, 190
hypersensitivity syndrome, 98, 145–146
cough reflex and, 99
inflammation, 69
muscles, palpation of, 101
nerve, superior, injection into, 182
reposturing, behavioral therapy and, 160
syndromes
history of, 97–98
symptoms of, 100
Laryngeal adductor response (LAR), 128
Laryngeal sensory neuropathy (LSN), 98
Laryngopharyngeal reflux disease (LPRD), cough and, 49
Laryngopharyngeal reflux (LPR), 6, 87
antireflux surgery, 86–87
chronic cough and, 46
CRS (Chronic rhinosinusitis) and, 44–45
described, 81
endoscopy and, 68–69
pepsin and, 175
Pepstatin A and, 88
PPI and, 88
refractory chronic cough and, 175
symptoms of, 65
Laryngopharynx, GERD and, 6, 87
Laryngoplasty, 191
Laryngoscope, flexible fiberoptic, visualization of larynx and, 10
Laryngoscopy, 153
flexible, 119
neurogenic cough and, 101, 101–103

Laryngospasm, 188
episodic, ILS and, 145
laryngeal hypersensitivity syndromes and, 100
Larynx
aspiration and, 67
chronic cough and, 117
hypersensitivity of, 192
pepsin and, 6
systematic disease of, 10
videostroboscopic evaluation, 153–154
visualization of, 10, 101–103
LCQ (Leicester Cough Questionnaire), 11, 147, 191
LDCT (Low-dose computerized tomography), 10
Left lateral decubitus position, reflux and, 72
Leicester Cough Questionnaire (LCQ), 11, 147, 191
LEMG (Laryngeal electromyography), 103
neurogenic cough and, 101
Lesions, proliferative, 135
Leukotriene modifiers, 30, 31–32
Leukotrienes, 22
Lidocaine, 127, 129
injection of, 182
Lifestyles, reflux and, 71–72
Likert scale, 11
Linx Reflux Management System, 74
Lipid-laden alveolar macrophage index (LLMI), 83
Liquid, coming out nose, 121
Lisinopril, 180
LLMI (Lipid-laden alveolar macrophage index), 83
Local anesthesia
cough reflex and, 3
LEMG and, 103
Long-acting beta agonists (LABAs), 30, 31
Low-dose computerized tomography (LDCT), 10
Lower
airway, upper airway relationships with, 44–45
bronchial, cigarette toxins and, 7
esophageal sphincter, TNE and, 129
gastrointestinal tract, scleroderma and, 135
LPR (Laryngopharyngeal reflux), 6
antireflux surgery, 86–87
chronic cough and, 46
CRS (Chronic rhinosinusitis) and, 44–45
described, 81
endoscopy and, 68–69
HRM and, 131
pepsin and, 175
Pepstatin A and, 88
PPI and, 88
refractory chronic cough and, 175
symptoms of, 65
LPRD (Laryngopharyngeal reflux disease), cough and, 49
LSN (Laryngeal sensory neuropathy), 98
Lung
collapsed, cough and, 2
volume, stretch receptors and, 3
cancer, tobacco and, 9
pathology, cough and, 187
Lymphocytes, T-helper, expressing Th2-type cytokines, 42

M

Macroaspiration, 67
Magnesium, Dead Sea salt and, 54
Magnetic ring procedures, 86
Malaise, chronic cough and, 13
Malignancy, cest roentgenogram and, 10
Malnutrition, dysplasia and, 118
Manual Assessment of Respiratory Motion (MARM), 162
Manuka honey, antimicrobial properties, 53–54
MARM (Manual Assessment of Respiratory Motion), 162
Mast cell mediators, 22
Maxillary sinus recirculation, 47
MBS (Barium swallow), 125–126
MCS (Multiple chemical sensitivity), 49

Medical history, 51
Medication trials, reflux and, 72
Medications, cough and, 68
Meditation, 190
Medtronic Inc., 70, 178
Membrane thickening, inflammation and, 43
Metasone, pregnancy and, 48
Metoclopramide, 72
MFR (Myofascial release), 160
MI (Motivational Interviewing), 157
Microaspiration, 67
Microbiocidal nitric oxide, Xylitol and, 53
Middle ear effusion, chronic cough and, 180
MII-pH, 71
  monitoring, 87
Mindfulness, 190
Mint, reflux and, 72
Mirror, visualization of larynx with, 102
Mitochondrial, damage, pepsin and, 6
Mometasone nasal spray, 53
Motivational Interviewing (MI), 157
Motor response, efferent vagal, 189
MTD (Muscle tension dysphonia), 145–146
  ILS and, 145
Mucosa, hypersecretion, 22
Mucosal eosinophilia, airway, 27
Mucous
  glands, swollen, 46
  plugging, 22
Mucus, hypersecretion, 43
Multichannel intraluminal impedance with dual pH (MII-pH) probe testing, 70, 82
Multiple chemical sensitivity (MCS), 49
Muscle
  habitual misuse of, 145
  palpable tension, 145
Muscle tension
  FHP and, 156
  SLPs observation of, 151–152
Muscle tension dysphonia (MTD), 145–146
Myofascial release (MFR), 160

N

NAR (Nonallergic rhinitis), 47
  asthma and, 42–45
    clinical relationship between, 42–43
  capsaicin and, 55
  described, 47
NARES (Nonallergic rhinitis with eosinophilia), 42, 47
Nasal
  bronchial reflex, 44
  dorsum, supratip crease on, 9
  drainage, purulent, 46
  endoscopy, 52
  obstruction, nasal to mouth breathing and, 45
  petrolatum packing, lower airway resistance and, 44
  polyposis, CAT and, 11
  polyps, CRS and, 41–42
  steroid spray, 53
  stimulus, with allergens, 44
  to mouth breathing, 45
Nasopharyngitis, 49
N-chlorotaurine (NCT), 54
NCT (N-chlorotaurine), 54
Neck, examination of, chronic cough and, 9
Neurogenic cough
  described, 97
  diagnosis of, 101
  history of, 97–98, 100–101
  laryngoscopy and, 101–103
  LEMG and, 103
  pathophysiology of, 99
  physical examination and, 100–101
  PVV and, 82
  stroboscopy and, 101–103
  treatment of, 104–108
    amitriptyline, 104–106
    baclofen, 108
    gabapentin, 106–108
    pregablin, 106–108
    tramadol, 108
  upper respiratory illness and, 100–101
Neuromodulating
  agents, 190
  medications, 180

Neuromodulator trials, 181
Neuromodulators, 97, 108–109
  chronic cough and, 104
  combined with speech therapy, 111
Neutrophilic asthma, 22
Nijmegen questionnaire (NQ), 162
Nissen fundoplication, 74, 83, 87, 182
Nitrates, reflux and, 72
NMDA (N-methyl-D-aspartate) receptors, 99
N-methyl-D-aspartate (NMDA) receptors, 99
Nodose ganglia, 3
Nonacid pepsin, 84
Nonacid reflux, 181
  etiology, 180
  LPR and, 87
Nonacidic high esophageal, 180
Nonallergic rhinitis (NAR)
  asthma and, 42–45
    clinical relationship between, 42–43
  capsaicin and, 55
  described, 47
Nonallergic rhinitis with eosinophilia (NARES), 42, 47
Nonasthmatic eosinophilic bronchitis, cough and, 68
Nonsmokers, GERD and, 66–67
Nose
  food/liquid coming out of, 121
  vasomotor rhinitis and, 47
NQ (Nijmegen questionnaire), 162

O

Obese asthma, 22
Objective reflux testing, 70–71, 72
Obstructive sleep apnea, 69
  reflux and, 71
Occupational asthma, 22
Odors
  asthma and, 23
  neurogenic cough and, 99
Odynophagia, 120–121
Oil red O, 83
Oral steroids, 30
Oropharyngeal dysphagia, aspiration and, 118
Osteomeatal complex disease, 48
Otolaryngologist, 40
  patient screening, 118–120
Oxitropium, 53
Oxymetazoline, 127, 129

P

$PACO_2$ (Alveolar carbon dioxide concentration), 162
  PVFMD and, 162
Pain, chronic. *See* Chronic pain
Pancreatic digestive enzymes, refluxate and, 65
Paradoxical vocal fold motion disorder (PVFMD), 145–146, 153, 156
  DB and, 160–161
  hyperventilation and, 162–163
  laryngoscopy and, 153
  voice therapy and, 158
Paranasal sinus
  computerized tomography (CAT) and, 11
  mucosal thickening, CAT and, 11
Passive smoke, exposure to, 9
Pathophysiology, interrelationship of upper and lower airway, 44–45
Patient
  education, SLPs and, 153
  flexible initial approach to, 174–178
  inventories, 11
Penetration
  chronic cough and, 117
  defined, 126
Pepsin
  in bronchoalveolar lavage (BAL), 82–83
  gastric reflux and, 6
  LPR and, 175
    mediated mucosal damage and, 86
  mediated reflux disease, 180
  as mediator of inflammatory diseases processes, 84–87
  reflux diagnosis and, 71
  refluxate and, 65
  as therapeutic target, 88
Pepsinogen, gastric reflux and, 6
Pepstatin A, 88

Periodic occurrence of laryngeal obstruction (POLO), 145
Persistent cough, childhood asthma and, 23
PFT (Pulmonary function test), 175
pH probe, double, LPR and, 11
Phantom irritation of the throat, 99
Pharyngeal
  manometry, 131
  muscle weakness, 131
  reflux, 180
    pepsin-induced, 146
Pharyngobronchial reflex, 46
Pharynx
  elevated laryngeal position in, 159
  sinonasal secretions and, 6
Phonation, chronic cough and, 143
Physical examination, 9–10
  pulmonary, 10
Physical irritants, rhinitis and, 47
Physiologic reflux, 175
Placebo nasal saline spray, 54
PND (Post nasal drip)
  chronic cough without evidence of, 46
  diagnosis of, 46–47
PNDS (Postnasal drip syndrome), 45–46
Pneumonia
  aspiration, 117
    dysplasia and, 118
Pneumothorax, cough and, 2
POLO (Periodic occurrence of laryngeal obstruction), 145
Positive bronchoconstrictor response, and cold air, 44
Post nasal drip (PND)
  chronic cough without evidence of, 46
  diagnosis of, 46–47
Posterior
  ethmoid disease, 48
  pharyngeal mucosa, cobblestoning of, 46
Postinfectious UACS, 47
Post-nasal drainage, dental pathology and, 49
  cough and, 187
Post-nasal drip syndrome (PNDS), 45–46
Postoperative
  care, saline irrigations and, 53
  infection, Manuka honey and, 53–54
Postprandial heartburn, GERD and, 66
Posture, SLPs and, 156–157
Postviral cough syndrome, inhaled anticholinergics and, 53
Postviral vagal neuropathy (PVVN), 47, 98, 117, 180
  symptoms of, 100
PPI (Proton-pump inhibitor), 72, 86, 176, 178
Preferred Practice Patterns for the Profession of Speech-Language Pathology, 119
Pregabalin, 106–108, 190
Pregnancy, rhinitis of, 47–48
Probes
  ComforTec LPR array, 70
  impedance/pH, 70
Progressive systemic sclerosis, dysplasia and, 135
Proinflammatory cytokine profile, 88
Prokinetics, 72
Proliferative lesions, 135
Prostaglandins, 22
Proteolytic digestive enzymes, gastric reflux and, 6
Proton-pump inhibitor (PPI), 72, 86, 88, 176, 178
Pruritus, AR and, 46
Pseudomonas aeruginosa, 53–54
Psychoeducational counseling, SLPs and, 157–158
Psychogenic cough, 189
Pulmonary function test (PFT), 175
Pulmonary physical examination, 10
Pulmonologist, 40
Purulent nasal drainage, 46
PVFMD (Paradoxical vocal fold motion disorder), 145–146, 153, 156
  DB and, 160–161
  hyperventilation and, 162–163
  laryngoscopy and, 153
  voice therapy and, 158
PVVN (Postviral vagal neuropathy), 47, 98, 117
  symptoms of, 100

Q

Quality of life
chronic cough and, 13–14
cough related, 145
Quick-relief bronchodilators, 28–29

R

Rab-9 endosome marker, 84
Radiesse voice gel, 192
Reactive Airway Disease, 5
Reckitt Benckiser, 181
Recreational drugs, vocal hygiene and, 147
Red wine, reflux and, 72
Reflective cough pathways, cortical influences in, 189–190
Reflux, 181–182
biomarkers in, 81–84
cough and, 187
cough stimulated by, 67
diagnosis of, 67–68
disease
cough/swallowing and, 117
HRM and, 131
diet and, 71–72
episodes of, 65
esophagitis, 69
GERD and, 66
lifestyles and, 71–72
medication trials and, 72
nonacid, 181
LPR and, 87
objective testing of, 72
pharyngeal, 180
pepsin-induced, 146
physiologic, 175
refractory, 44, 74
surgery, 73–74
testing, objective of, 70–71
workup, 175
Reflux Finding Score (RFS), 10, 65, 82
Reflux Symptom Index (RSI), 65, 82, 147, **151**
Refluxate, 65
Refractory
chronic cough, 14, 67, 183, 187
antireflux surgery and, 182
Botox injections and, 192
diagrammatic approach to, 178
LPR and, 175
SLPs and, 176
patients, 175
reflux, 44, 74
Refractory chronic cough wheel, 178, **179**
Regurgitation,
GERD and, 66
surgery and, 73
Remodeled airways, 22
Rentgenogram, chest, 10
Respiration, chronic cough and, 143
infections, bronchoconstriction and, 22
retraining, SLPs and, 157
Respiratory Technology Corp., 175
Restech® Dx-pH probe, 175
Retrosternal chest pain, GERD and, 66
RFS (Reflux Finding Score), 10, 65, 82
Rhinitis, 40
allergic
asthma and, 41
described, 46
intranasal hypertonic saline and, 54
management of, 49
saline irrigations and, 53
medicamentosa, 47–48
hormonal, 47–48
nonallergic
asthma and, 42–45
capsaicin and, 55
of pregnancy, 47–48
Rhinitis rhinorrhea
AR and, 46
symptoms of, 47
Rhinosinusitis, 40
chronic
clinical relationship between, 43–44
management of, 49
eosinophilic, 41
Ribs, broken, cough and, 2
Rigid Hopkins rod laryngoscopes, visualization of larynx with, 102

Rigid transoral laryngoscopy, visualization of larynx with, 102
RSI (Reflux Symptom Index), 65, 82, 147, **151**

S

SABAs (Short-acting beta-agonists), acute bronchoconstriction and, 28
Saline irrigations, 53
Salmeterol Multicenter Asthma Research Trial (SMART), 31
Salute, allergic, 10
Sarcoidosis, 10, 69
S-A-W (Systematic disease of the larynx), sarcoidosis and, 10
Scalene, FHP and, 156
Scleroderma
 dysplasia and, 135
 gastrointestinal tracts and, 135
Sclerosis, progressive systemic, dysplasia and, 135
SEBQ (Self-Evaluation of Breathing Questionnaire), 162
Self-Evaluation of Breathing Questionnaire (SEBQ), 162
Sensorimotor cortex, 190
Septoplasty, 175
Serum biomarkers, 27–28
Shiners, allergic, 10
Short-acting beta-agonists (SABAs), acute bronchoconstriction and, 28
Shortness of breath, cough-variant asthma, 21
Silent
 laughing, 156
 PND, 46
 UACS, 51
Silica, lower airway resistance and, 44
Sinonasal
 disease, 45–49
 drainage, aspiration of, 45
Sino-Nasal Outcome Test 20 (SNOT-20), Xylitol and, 53
Sinus surgery
 endoscopic, CRS and, 44
 saline irrigations and, 53
Sleep
 apnea, 69
  reflux and, 72
 chronic cough and, 13
SLN (Superior laryngeal nerve), block, 192–193
SLPs (Speech-language pathologist), 143–144
 case history and, 147–151
 chronic cough and, 144–145
 clinician observations, 151–152
 cough control strategies, 155
 functional measurements by, 152–153
 inclusion/exclusion criteria, 146–147
 laryngeal deconstriction techniques, 156
 pathophysiology of, 118
 patient education, 153
 posture and, 156–157
 psychoeducational counseling, 157–158
 refractory chronic cough and, 176
 respiratory retraining, 157
 speech pathology intervention and, 153–154
 suppression/distracting techniques, 155–156
 vocal hygiene and, 154–155
 voice therapy, 158
SMART (Salmeterol Multicenter Asthma Research Trial), 31
Smoke, exposure to passive, 9
Smokers cough, 7, 9
Smoking
 bronchitis and, 7
 cough and, 45, 49, 187
 reflux and, 72
 vocal hygiene and, 147
Smooth muscle
 constriction, stretch receptors and, 3
 hyperplasia, 22
 hypertrophy, 22
Sneezing, AR and, 46
SNOT-20 (Sino-Nasal Outcome Test 20), Xylitol and, 53
Sodium alginate suspensions, 72
Sodium hyaluronate, 54

Speech-language pathologist (SLPs), 143–144
case history and, 147–151
chronic cough and, 144–145
clinician observations, 151–152
cough control strategies, 155
functional measurements by, 152–153
inclusion/exclusion criteria, 146–147
laryngeal deconstriction techniques, 156
pathophysiology of, 118
patient education, 154
posture and, 156–157
psychoeducational counseling, 157–158
refractory chronic cough and, 176
respiratory retraining, 157
speech pathology intervention and, 153–154
suppression/distracting techniques, 155–156
vocal hygiene and, 154–155
voice therapy, 158
Speech pathology intervention, 153–154
Speech Pathology Management of Chronic Refractory Cough and Related Disorders, 146
Speech therapy, 190
combined with neuromodulators, 111
goals of, 153–154
Sphincter dysfunction, 182
Sputum, quality and quantity produced, 52
Staphylococcus aureus, 53–54
Stenosis, subglottic, LPR and, 65
Sternocleidomastoid (SCM), FHP and, 156
Steroid inhalers, 175
Steroids, 175
injection of, 182
nasal spray, 53
oral, 30
Stomach, TNE and, 129
Stretch receptors, 3, **4**
Stricture, TNE and, 129
Stridor, chronic cough and, 143, 145
Stroboscopic light, 153
Stroboscopy, neurogenic cough and, 101–103
Subepithelial
edema, 43
fibrosis, 22
Subglottic stenosis, LPR and, 65
Subglottis, Wegener's in, 10
Suggestion therapy, 190
Sulcus vocalis, 192
Superior laryngeal nerve (SLN)
block, block, 192–193
injection into, 182
Supine reflux, GERD and, 66
Supraglottic
constriction, 158
larynx, sarcoidosis and, 10
Supraglottis, sarcoid in, 10
Supratip crease, on nasal dorsum, 9
Surfactants, 54
Surgery, 190–193
Swallowing
anesthesia and, 127
chronic cough and, 117, 143
clinical evaluation of, 120–125
examination and, 118
Symptom scores, eosinophile count and, 43
Symptomatic cough, 117
Syncope, cough and, 2
Systematic disease of the larynx (S-A-W), sarcoidosis and, 10
Systemic amplification, theory of, 45

T

Tachyphylaxis, to bronchoprotective effect, 28
TCA (Tricyclic antidepressant), 104
anticholinergic effects of, 106
Th2 lymphocytes, cytokines and, 43
T-helper
inflammation, 43
lymphocytes, expressing Th2-type cytokines, 42
Therapy, 190
Thermoplasty, bronchial, 32–33, 182–183

Thoracic airway, vagal afferents and, **4**
Thornwaldt's cyst, 49
Throat
  breathing, relaxed, 156
  clearing, 69
    LPR and, 65
    neurogenic cough and, 101
  phantom irritation of, 99
Tic cough, 189
Time-synchronized audio, 71
Tiotropium, 53
TNE (Transnasal esophagoscopy), 128–130
Tobacco, exposure to, physical examination and, 9
Tomography, low-dose computerized, 10
Tooth, enamel degradation, GERD and, 66
Topical
  anesthetic, FEES and, 127
  capsaicin, 55
Tramadol, 190–191
Transnasal esophagoscopy (TNE), 128–130
Transreticular Golgi (TRG), 84
Trapezius muscles, FHP and, 156
Treatment approaches, 190–193
TRG (Transreticular Golgi), 84
TRG-46, 84
Triamcinolone spray, 54
Tricyclic antidepressant (TCA), 104
  anticholinergic effects of, 106
TRPV1 receptors, 189
Tryptase, 22

U

UACS (Upper airway cough syndrome), 6–7, 45–47
  cough and, 49
  defined, American College of Chest Physicians, 7
  postinfectious, 47
  silent, 51
  treatment of, 52
UES (Upper esophageal sphincter), 126, 175
Ulcers, Manuka honey and, 53–54
Unified airway, 180
  model, 40–42, 45
  upper and lower airway relationship, 40–42
Upper aerodigestive tract, aspiration and, 67
Upper airway
  cough and, 39
  directed treatments, 55
  lower airway relationships with, 44–45
Upper airway cough syndrome (UACS), 6–7, 45–47
  cough and, 49
  postinfectious, 47
  silent, 51
  treatment of, 52
Upper airway disorders, linked to chronic cough, 145–146
Upper airway tract
  infections, asthma and, 23
  sensitivity to reflux, 86
Upper cranial neuropathies, vagal neuropathy and, 101
Upper esophageal sphincter (UES), 126, 175
Upper gastrointestinal tract, scleroderma and, 135
Upper respiratory infection (URI), 53, 100–101, 187
  acute viral, 47
  inhaled anticholinergics and, 53
  PVVN and, 117
Upper respiratory infections, cough and, 187
Upper respiratory tract
  clinical examination of, 51–52
  neurogenic cough and, 100–101
Upper respiratory tract infection (URTI), cough and, 144
URI (Upper respiratory infection), 100–101, 187
  acute viral, 47
  inhaled anticholinergics and, 53
  PVVN (Postviral vagal neuropathy), 117
  unhailed anticholinergics and, 53

Urinary incontinence, cough and, 2
URTI (Upper respiratory tract infection), cough and, 144

V

Vagal
afferents, 4, **4**
nerve dysfunction, 100
neuropathy, 98
upper cranial neuropathies and, 101
Vagotomy, cough reflex and, 3
Vagus nerve, 182
dysplasia and, 117
Vasomotor rhinitis, 47
Venous congestion, 9–10
VFSS (Videofluoroscopic swallow study), 176, 181
diverticula and, 131–132
dysphagia and, 125–126
VHI-10 (Voice Handicap Index-10-Item), 147, **149**
Videofluoroscopic swallow study (VFSS), 176, 181
diverticula and, 131–132
dysphagia and, 125–126
Videostroboscopic evaluation, of larynx, 153
Videostroboscopy, 69
Viral
etiology, acute cough and, 1
illness, ILS and, 98, 145
inflammation, neuropeptides and, 99
URI, 47
Vocal activities, vocal hygiene and, 147
Vocal cords
dysfunction, 145–146
sarcoidosis and, 10
Vocal fold
augmentation, 191
closure, 182
paresis, 192
PVV and, 82
Vocal hygiene, 147
SLPs and, 154–155
Vocal-use habits, SLPs observation of, 151–152
Voice assessment, 152
Voice gel, Radiesse, 192
Voice Handicap Index-10(VHI-10), 147, **149**
Voice therapist, chronic cough and, 181
Voice therapy, SLPs and, 158
Volitional cough, 4
Vomiting, GERD and, 66

W

Water
swallow tests, predicting aspiration risk with, 119
vocal hygiene and, 147
Wegener's deposits, sarcoidosis and, 10
Weight loss, reflux and, 71
Wheezing
asthma and, 5
childhood, 23
cough-variant asthma, 21
expiratory, 10
Widdicombe receptors, 3, **4**
Wine, reflux and, 72

X

Xylitol, 53

Z

Zenker's diverticulum, 131–132
Zwitterionic surfactant, 54